After Brain Injury: Tools for Living

A Step-by-Step Guide

for Caregivers and Survivors

J. Lynne Mann with Michael Rossiter

Copyright © 2003 J. Lynne Mann and Michael Rossiter

All rights reserved. No part of this publication may be reproduced without express written permission of the publisher, except in the case of brief quotations embodied in critical articles or reviews. Purchasers of this book have our permission to reproduce the worksheets.

National Library of Canada Cataloguing in Publication

Mann, J. Lynne, 1949-
After brain injury : tools for living : a step-by-step guide for caregivers & survivors / J. Lynne Mann, Michael Rossiter.

ISBN 1-894694-25-2

1. Brain--Wounds and injuries--Patients--Rehabilitation.
2. Brain damage--Patients--Rehabilitation.
3. Brain--Wounds and injuries--Psychological aspects.
 I. Rossiter, Michael, 1944-
 II. Title.

RC387.5.M35 2003   617.4'8103   C2003-905243-5

Editing by Suzanne Bastedo
Book design by Fiona Raven
Cover design by Michael Rossiter
Illustrations by Teresa Waclawik

First Printing January 2004
Printed in Hong Kong

Granville Island Publishing
Suite 212–1656 Duranleau
Vancouver, BC, Canada V6H 3S4
Tel 604-688-0320 Toll-free 1-877-688-0320
www.granvilleislandpublishing.com

Granville Island
Publishing

Can be ordered at www.livingafterbraininjury.com
or by telephone at 1-866-520-3468

Disclaimer: This book represents the thoughts and programs developed by J. Lynne Mann, Registered Psychologist, and supported by the experiences of Michael Rossiter, the father of a brain-injury survivor and advocate for such survivors. The information given in it is not intended to be taken as a replacement for medical advice.

Table of Contents

Acknowledgments 8
In the Beginning 9

Introduction 11
Why read this book? 11
How far can you go in recovery? 12
What is psychological recovery? 14
Chapter summaries 15

1 Looking at the Psychological Self — 19

Learning goals for this chapter 19
Who's responsible for this next stage of recovery? 20
Why is knowing yourself important? 21
Looking at the Psychological Self 23
    The Social Self 26
    The Real Self 27
When the Social Self and Real Self don't communicate well ... 29

2 Having Inner Conversations Again — 37

Learning goals for this chapter	37
Why is it important to have inner conversations again?	38
Willpower and willingness	39
Keeping a journal	44
Contacting your Social Self and your Real Self	46
Understanding denial as a stopper to inner conversations	48
Dealing with your survivor's brain-based denial	53
Stop-Still-Think (SST) Instructional Aid	57
Dealing with your own self-based denial	59
Making inner conversations safe	65

3 Recovering Emotionally — 69

Learning goals for this chapter	69
What does it mean to recover emotionally?	71
What is trauma?	73
Core issues in Emotional Recovery	75
Trauma Roles: Victim - Rescuer - Persecutor	77
Letting go of trauma roles	80
The Five-Stage Emotional Recovery Model	84
Stage 1 – Daily Survival	87
Stage 2 – Re-Identification	90
Stage 3 – Dealing with Core Issues	95
Stage 4 – Integration	98
Stage 5 – Genesis	99
Issues in Emotional Recovery	102

4 Thinking in New Ways — 103

Learning goals for this chapter	103
The Brain and How It Affects Thinking	107
The Brain's Jobs	108
The Frontal Lobe as a Conductor	109

Strategies and Tools for Learning Six Thinking Skills	110
(1) Setting goals	111
(2) Making decisions effectively	114
(3) Doing a task analysis	116
(4) Solving problems	120
(5) Planning projects	124
(6) Managing time	127

5 Changing Behavior — 131

Learning goals for this chapter	131
Why change behavior?	133
What Works When Changing Behavior	134
Stages in Learning New Behavior	136
Three Models for Changing Behavior	138
Mastery Model	139
Five-Stage Goal-Setting Model	140
Task-Analysis Model	150
An Example of Changing Behavior: Changing Anger	153
Setting a weekly goal	154
Identifying your anger style and trigger conditions	154
Measuring anger	156
Reviewing goals	157
Concluding Remarks	159
The Pocket Guide: Key Points Related to each Chapter	160

Resources — 161

Worksheets from All Chapters	162
Further Resources Available	186

Author Biographies 188

Acknowledgments

J. Lynne Mann

This book, the Pocket Guide, the TOM System, the coaching/support line and the Facilitator's Guide happened only because we had a team of supportive, committed and excited people gathered about the planning table.

First, thanks to Mike Rossiter and to John Wright. Mike, with his never-ending commitment to developing educational resources for families, kept me going when my enthusiasm waned in the midst of all the work. He knows the needs of families in a way I do not. John, our Sales and Marketing partner, brings a wealth of knowledge and giving to the challenge of getting the word out about the book and other educational products.

Gisela Theurer, coach and President of GMT Consultants, joined us as we began to think about how we could offer ongoing support and help. Thanks, Gisela, for your clarity about the type of helping that coaching represents.

To Tina, Keith, Tim, Cherie, Lisa, Val and Murray, thanks for volunteering to test out changes to the TOM System. Your help clarified my thinking.

To the friends, colleagues and clients who are ever patient with my limitations and questions about what are incredibly complex subjects (the brain, being human, growing, recovery, and change), thank you.

John Saremba offered some of his ideas, which were incorporated in the TOM System. Thanks, John. Finally, thanks to Jo Blackmore, Fiona Raven, Teresa Waclawik, Peter Breikss and Suzanne Bastedo for all your instrumental ideas. And to Lisa because she is Lisa.

In The Beginning

J. Lynne Mann

When I was 11, I began to have seizures and was eventually diagnosed as having epilepsy. My young teenagehood was marked by visits to neurologists who would ask questions and occasionally change medications. Being the person who would one day become a psychologist, I wondered about the fact that most of my seizures happened during periods of stress. When I asked about this relationship between stress and seizures, I was met by silence. I did not understand at that age that a medical professional might not have such a body of knowledge.

Young but sure of myself (what is youth for if not to be sure!), I resolved to one day write a book about stress and the meaning of being a person with epilepsy.

Years later, the book written as a requirement of my graduate program, I went on to discover the world of rehabilitation. Rehabilitation and recovery became visible to me as I began my professional career. Working with adults with neurological disabilities has remained my focus.

Working in the field of rehabilitation, I discovered the 80-20 rule: 80 per cent of the time spent face-to-face with our clients was spent in assessment, 20 per cent of the time was devoted to treatment. This bothered me. I saw that my profession, which I love, was becoming inaccessible to people wanting help to get better. Twenty years ago, I left public practice to develop treatment programs that focus on the Psychological Self, the emotional recovery process and return to work.

Practical help, not psychotherapy alone, became the focus of my private practice and the work we do within my company. Whether we work on return to work or on emotional recovery, people are looking for practical ways to manage their thinking, their emotional lives and their behavior.

Then Mike and I began having lunch. . . .

Michael Rossiter

It was 3:00 a.m. on November 4, 1995, when we received the phone call. The voice on the line was trying to find a comforting way to tell us that our son, age 21, had been in a terrible accident and may not live much longer. I cannot describe how helpless it feels to listen to those words from a total stranger and from a distance of 500 air miles away. My father was a policeman and always said it was a duty every cop dreaded. Now I was the recipient of that kind of call.

My son eventually came out of the coma in the hospital and, after three months of struggling through rehab to learn the basics of eating and motor skills, he said his first words. I will always remember them: "I love you, Dad." He moved on from the hospital to a rehab center, where they worked on his movement and cognitive skills. This work was successful enough to get him placed in a group home to help with the move to semi-dependent living in the community.

For me the years have seemed to move by quickly since my son's accident, and many changes have taken place. I sold my business interests and home in the north, and moved to Vancouver to be close to my son. My first wife and I were divorced five years ago. Like me, she continues to be a strong advocate for our son. Two years ago I was diagnosed with cancer and underwent six months of chemotherapy. Last year I married a wonderful woman, who has been very supportive.

It has been a rocky, eight-year journey for my son as well as for our family — one filled with frustration, determination and everyday struggles. My son uses an electric wheelchair as his legs, and he battles daily with his memory and social skills. He is a proud man who works hard to live independently in the community. He is truly my hero.

This road will never end for survivors, families and caregivers until people with brain injuries are accepted as a part of our communities. People with brain injuries deserve the same respect and opportunities as anyone else. And to that end we need to continue to advocate for our loved ones.

Mike Rossiter

Introduction

Why read this book?

This book looks at each of the four areas of psychological recovery and provides step-by-step methods and tools for each area. The information here will help you in your recovery and give you ways to help your loved one, too. In this book, you will:

- be exposed to new ideas about becoming more self-aware, recovering emotionally, thinking in new ways, and changing behavior
- learn new methods and tools for solving problems
- practice these methods and tools by doing worksheets
- be inspired to try out these methods and skills in everyday situations
- develop your ability to remember these ideas on your own

Sometimes I lie awake at night, and I ask, "Where have I gone wrong?" Then a voice says to me, "This is going to take more than one night."

— Charlie Brown

This book is one of the *After Brain Injury: Tools for Living* system of educational products designed to help caregivers and survivors in the hard work of recovery from the trauma of brain injury. You may use this book alone, or with the other educational products.

This book is based on the belief that it is not only the survivor of brain injury who needs to recover, but also the survivor's family and friends — and especially you, the caregiver. Each chapter is designed to guide you as a caregiver in your psychological recovery after the loss and upheaval of your loved one's brain injury.

In each chapter you will find worksheets and instructional aids to use as you work through your own recovery. So that you will also have this material to use as you help your loved one in her/his recovery, the Resources section at the end of the book has blank copies of all the worksheets contained within the chapters. In the Resources section you will also find a list of Internet resources you can access.

How far can you go in recovery?

Life after brain injury brings a wide range of changes. Your loved one has experienced many changes — in skills, thinking, emotional control, and identity. You and the rest of your family have had your own set of reactions to this traumatic event: confusion, grief, and changes in self-awareness, emotions, thinking, and behavior. You might even be involved in litigation, which many families identify as a stress that can continue for years.

Most of the help you receive will be offered and provided early in the physical recovery process. Your loved one might

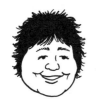

Lynne says...
The chapters in this book are for you, the caregiver. Like most caregivers, your first concern is probably not you, but the survivor you care for and about. Although much of the information here applies to both you and the survivor, it focuses on you. As the caregiver, you need to start recovering psychologically before you can help your loved one.

stay in the hospital for a long time or a short time — or not at all. Life after that remains a journey where you and your loved one will be guided by your own best resources. You probably already realize that resources to help you and your loved one with psychological recovery are hard, if not impossible, to locate. Many caregivers and survivors find that their learning and growth end too soon, not because they have reached their maximum levels of recovery, but because they have reached the limits of their own ideas and experience.

This book will give you new ideas and experience, but it's not the only thing you need. How far you — and your loved one — go in your recovery will be affected by:

- your willingness to learn new things

- your patience and your determination to stick to this new learning when the going gets tough

- the limits you are able to discover within yourself (and everyone has limits)

- your psychological need for safety as you grow

By opening this book, you have already shown the key attitude you will need for as full a recovery as possible — an attitude of willingness to learn new things. While it sometimes seems hard, you will learn more by stepping outside your comfort zone into the unknown than by staying where you are. By using this book, you will be taking small steps toward change in a safe and positive way.

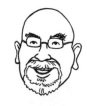

Mike says... **For the first stages of brain injury, there were all kinds of supports and services available. As soon as we moved into the community, funding dried up. So did services and social acceptance. Now I know that many people did not even get these first funded services.**

Of course, making changes means that you have to be ready to accept some risk. As you read this book and try the methods and tools presented, remember that you are in control of how many changes you try to make and how often you take some small risks in doing so.

If you have a learning buddy, you might enjoy the journey more. Ask a friend or trusted person to join you in working through this book. The methods and tools presented here do not apply only to people with brain injuries and their caregivers. Anyone could find these methods and tools useful in their lives.

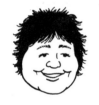

Lynne says... There are many people and places to go to find information and support soon after a brain injury. Later on, these supports fade. Mike and I wrote this to help caregivers later, after the supports fade.

What is psychological recovery?

Physical recovery and healing is the first thing everyone focuses on after brain injury. You and your loved one have needed courage and determination to face the tasks of physical recovery.

Before you start this book, take some time to appreciate all that you and your loved one have done to get this far in recovery. The hours, days and months spent as your loved one regained physical skills gave you both important lessons in motivation, willpower, and clear results. You will use these valuable lessons again and again to support your continued healing and growth.

This stage, after your loved one has started to recover and heal physically, is when you both might be asking: What's next? For most survivors and caregivers, what's next is recovering psychologically. Psychological recovery involves four main areas of recovery: self-awareness (also called recovering the Psychological Self), emotions, thinking, and behavior.

These four areas of recovery will become very important as you work at finding a place in your community where you feel valued and where you can contribute, whether this involves being a friend, an intimate companion, a worker, a teacher, or a learner. The four areas are reflected in this book. Chapters 1 and 2 help you understand the Psychological Self, the part of you that needs to recover after the loss and upheaval of brain injury. Chapter 3 shows you ways of understanding and guiding your emotional recovery. Chapters 4 and 5 give you methods and tools for thinking in new ways and changing behavior after brain injury.

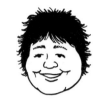

Lynne says…
Our brain controls everything we do, think and feel. This book strips the physical part out and works on the non-physical parts of getting better.

Chapter summaries

What follows is a brief introduction to each chapter.

Chapters 1 and 2

Since this is your book, you can start at any point in the book. However, it is a good idea to start with Chapter 1, "Looking at the Psychological Self," because psychological recovery depends very much on being self-aware.

Like many things in life, becoming self-aware requires constant learning. When you were a child, you had a picture of yourself that you carried inside you. That picture looks very different now, at this stage of your life. You can't yet know how you will see yourself next year or ten years from now. Your awareness of self will change with living and with your staying open to the lessons in life. Chapter 1 helps you picture your Psychological Self as it is now, understand it, and see what it does. Chapter 1 answers the question: Who am I, right now?

With awareness of the Psychological Self comes knowledge about how to get started on psychological recovery. Chapter 2, "Having Inner Conversations Again," focuses on the second important step in becoming more self-aware: learning to have conversations with your Psychological Self. The chapter also helps you understand denial, a main stopper to these conversations.

These first two chapters and the exercises they contain will help you understand that:

- Your relationship to yourself is central to all your psychological growth and healing.
- How you communicate within yourself affects how you communicate with others.
- Your Psychological Self manages your feelings, thoughts and actions.

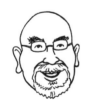

Mike says ... Even now, after eight years, I still sometimes feel guilty when I want to focus on me, and my whole family.

Chapter 3

Each brain injury is unique. This uniqueness results from two facts: (1) all people are unique, and (2) the brain is so complex that even similar injuries can have different impacts. It is also true that emotional recovery is predictable — most people have similar basic issues, or core issues, and go through the same five stages of recovery. Most people also take on trauma roles in hard times, sometimes acting as a victim, sometimes as a persecutor, and sometimes as a rescuer.

Chapter 3, "Recovering Emotionally," helps you make the predictability of emotional recovery work for you. It helps you identify where you are in emotional recovery and gives you tools that can heal. Chapter 3 will help you understand:

- your current core issues
- the five stages of emotional recovery
- your trauma roles

Chapters 4 and 5

Chapters 4 and 5 focus on two things that affect most survivors of brain injury and their caregivers: changes in thinking and behavior. These chapters will increase your understanding of the changes in thinking and behavior after brain injury and show you ways to help your loved one. In the process, you will probably find that you are changing your own ways of thinking and behaving, too.

Chapter 4, "Thinking in New Ways," reflects the fact that living with someone who has a brain injury usually means living with changed thinking skills. Memory, attention, judgment, problem-solving, decision-making, and impulse control are all affected.

Chapter 4 will help you understand:

- what parts of the brain are usually affected by a brain injury
- what strategies and tools you can use for helping your loved one learn important thinking skills

Chapter 5, "Changing Behavior," is the final chapter of the book. It focuses on changing behavior that has been affected

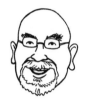

Mike says...
I believe that what you are about to learn is the place we all need to start. Take it one step at a time, in the order we present the chapters. The message will become more clear. One part will help you do other parts.

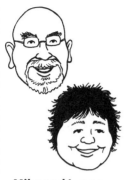

**Mike and Lynne say...
Remember that you can write in this book. It's yours. You can tear off a page, bend a corner, or highlight words. Feel free to use it as you like. It is your book. We put wide margins in this book for you. And...you can write or phone and ask for more detail.**

by brain injury. Placing this chapter last was done deliberately, so that you have the chance to work through the topics covered in the earlier chapters. By the time you have reached this chapter, you understand your Psychological Self better, you have started having inner conversations again, you know that emotional recovery happens in predictable stages, and you know that you can practice thinking skills that affect your behavior. You are now ready to tackle behavior change realistically.

Chapter 5 looks at what works when changing behavior and provides you with three models for changing behavior. Each model shows a different way of working with your loved one or yourself to change behavior. This chapter will help you understand:

- stages in learning new behavior
- what models work best at certain stages
- ways of breaking down learning goals into small, manageable pieces

Throughout this book, you will see this icon. It refers to key points that will be summarized and included in **The Pocket Guide**. After reading the book you are holding, you may need only The Pocket Guide when helping your loved one. The Guide is meant as a compact reference tool for you, your survivor, and for other caregivers.

1 Looking at the Psychological Self

Learning goals for this chapter

This chapter focuses on an important first step in getting to know yourself again — looking at your Psychological Self. The Psychological Self is the part of you in charge of psychological recovery. This chapter helps you picture your Psychological Self, understand it, and see what it does. The information here will help you in your recovery and give you ways to help your loved one.

In this chapter you will:

- be introduced to the idea of the Psychological Self
- learn what the Psychological Self does to keep you safe and well
- look at what happens when the parts of the Psychological Self don't communicate well (Chapter 2 will show you ways of having those inner conversations again)

After Brain Injury: Tools for Living
A Step-by-Step Guide for Caregivers and Survivors

Introduction

Who's responsible for this next stage of recovery?

When your loved one went through physical recovery, others led the way. Now you may be asking who is responsible for this next step in recovery — psychological healing and growth. The answer is:

You are.

Your loved one is responsible for his or her own recovery. You can help your loved one's recovery, though, if your recovery is also underway.

What does being responsible for yourself mean?

You can't take charge of yourself until you know who you are, now. That what's being responsible means.

Knowing yourself means being able to look inside yourself to see how you think and feel, then using this knowledge to understand yourself and the world around you. Knowing yourself helps you see and understand your own thoughts, feelings, values, hopes, dreams, goals, and actions. You have probably heard other words for knowing yourself, such as self-awareness, insight, self-identity, or self-reflection.

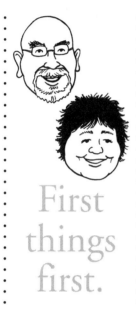

First things first.

Mike and Lynne say … First things first. Remember what is said in airplane safety instructions: 'Put the mask on yourself before you assist others.'

Chapter 1: Looking at the Psychological Self
Introduction

Survivors of brain injury often lose the ability to look inside themselves and see how they think and feel. As the caregiver of a survivor of brain injury, you have also experienced many changes in your life. You may also find your ability to look inside yourself affected. Luckily, like many other things you have learned, this ability can and often does return when you have a chance to relearn and to practice.

Why is knowing yourself important?

Getting back the ability to look inside yourself and become more aware of yourself is an important step for you and your loved one, too. Without the ability to look inside yourself and become more aware of yourself, you might not be able to move successfully through the other stages of recovery, from experiencing and expressing feelings, to thinking in new ways, to changing behavior. You might become stuck. Throughout your life, you might find yourself facing the same issues over and over again, without healing or growth.

Other words for knowing yourself:

self-awareness

insight

self-identity

self-reflection

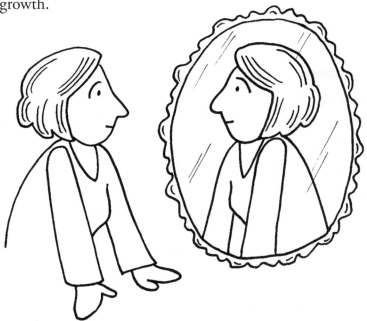

After Brain Injury: Tools for Living
A Step-by-Step Guide for Caregivers and Survivors

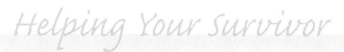

Knowing Yourself

Knowing yourself means being able to look inside yourself to see how you think and feel, then using this knowledge to understand yourself and the world around you. Knowing yourself helps you see and understand your own thoughts, feelings, values, hopes, dreams, goals, and actions.

You have probably heard other words for knowing yourself, such as insight, self-awareness, self-identity, or self-reflection. You can probably come up with other names.

Many survivors of brain injury say that they have lost their sense of identity, their sense of themselves. In truth, they don't know themselves any more. You might feel this way, too.

Many survivors who have gone through psychological recovery say that these are the best ways to get to know yourself again:

- make the decision to know yourself better

- try to stay positive

- choose a safe place and a safe person for asking questions

- find out about the Psychological Self

- gather tools that help you learn about your own Psychological Self

- practice what you learn

Looking at the Psychological Self

This chapter is designed to help you start looking at your Psychological Self in a new way, with recognition and appreciation. As you explore your Psychological Self, you will gather ideas and tools for healing and growing, for you and for your loved one, too.

What is the Psychological Self?

Healing and growing that lasts for life has a lot to do with the Psychological Self. This is the part of you that can bring about changes in feelings, thinking, and behavior. The Psychological Self has three main parts:

- an outer Social Self, which has the jobs of protecting and communicating

- an inner Real Self, which has many jobs, including growing, creating, interpreting wants and needs, finding a safe place for certain feelings

- the automatic protection mechanism of denial, which has the job of protecting you from too much worry (more about this later)

Others can easily see your physical self. They can see the color of your skin, the wrinkles in your forehead, and the clothes you wear. It's easy to understand the idea of physical self because it can be seen.

The Psychological Self is a much more difficult idea to understand because it can't be seen. But...what if someone

Lynne says ... Since 1987, I've used the Psychological Self approach in my emotional recovery groups for survivors and families. Many caregivers and survivors have found this approach very helpful for their recovery. I'm happy to share it with you here.

After Brain Injury: Tools for Living
A Step-by-Step Guide for Caregivers and Survivors

The Psychological Self

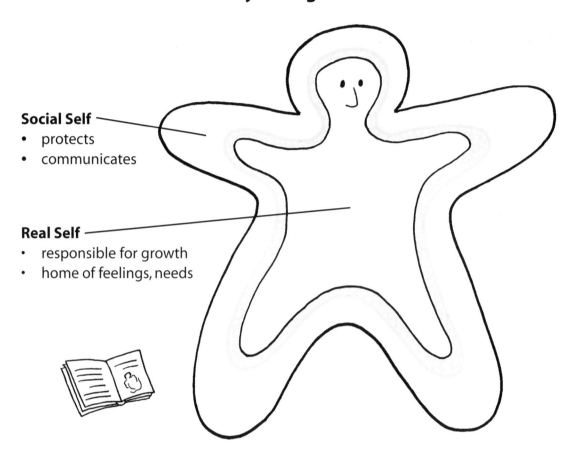

Social Self
- protects
- communicates

Real Self
- responsible for growth
- home of feelings, needs

drew a picture of the Psychological Self? The picture above shows what the Psychological Self could look like.

Now take a few moments to draw a picture of your own Psychological Self. What does it look like right now? On the following page you will see this worksheet:

- (1-1) A Picture of My Psychological Self

Don't worry about whether you are an artist or not. Let the picture describe yourself — both the inner and the outer parts, the parts other people see and the parts they don't.

W 1–1

Chapter 1: Looking at the Psychological Self
What is the Psychological Self?

A Picture of My Psychological Self

Here is where you can draw a picture of your Psychological Self.

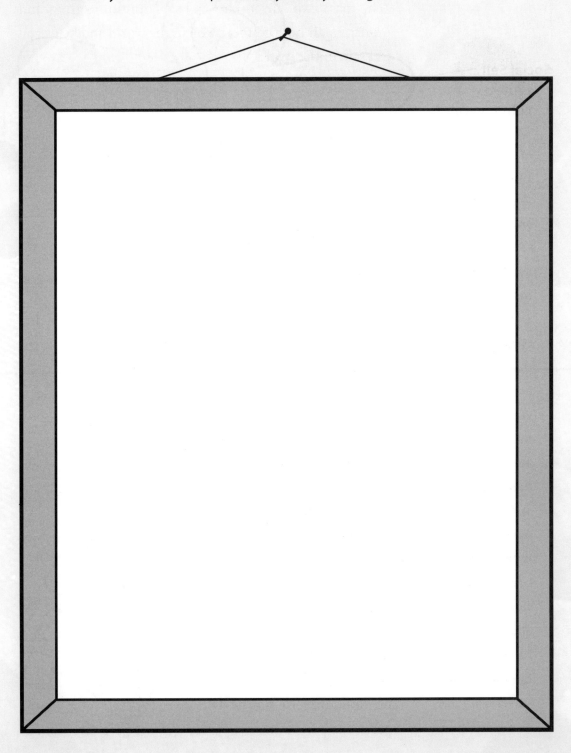

After Brain Injury: Tools for Living
A Step-by-Step Guide for Caregivers and Survivors

The Social Self

The Social Self, the larger, outside part of the Psychological Self, has two important jobs: communicating and protecting. It both connects you to the world and helps you feel safe in the world.

To do these jobs, the Social Self looks in two directions:

- toward the outside world, gathering information about it, taking part in it, and making judgments about your safety

- toward the inner, Real Self, to see how you feel about yourself and the outside world

The Social Self is the part of the Psychological Self that other people usually notice first. It's the part of the Psychological Self that communicates with other people. Your Social Self doesn't only use words to communicate. It also uses facial expressions, such as frowning or smiling, and body language, such as folding your arms or jiggling your foot.

Everyone needs a strong Social Self to interact with others. The strong Social Self pays attention to the outside world. But the Social Self can't pay attention only to that outside world. The Social Self also needs to pay attention to the Real Self's needs.

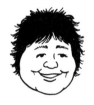

Lynne says . . . By the end of this chapter, you will be able to help the survivor with both your head and your heart. With your thoughtful, informed head, you can teach the survivor about the Psychological Self and how to use it in recovery. With your heart, because you care for and about the survivor, you can support the survivor in your own special way.

The Real Self

The Real Self is the inner and smaller part of the Psychological Self. The Real Self holds those parts of yourself that you feel are special, private, and vulnerable.

Be yourself — who else is better qualified?

FRANK J. GIBLIN II

The Real Self has a number of special jobs:

- to make sure that the Social Self knows what feels safe and unsafe

- to hold feelings and needs

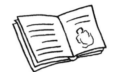

- to create solutions to problems

- to make good decisions about actions to take

- to give permission to try new things

- to guide impulsive behavior: actions taken very quickly without planning or thinking

Think about what the Real Self does for you:

1. Think of a recent time when you had an important decision to make. Write about how your Real Self helped:
   _____
   _____

2. Now think of a time when your deepest wishes or feelings found expression. Maybe you felt so safe, you risked self-disclosure. Write a short description here:
   _____
   _____

After Brain Injury: Tools for Living
A Step-by-Step Guide for Caregivers and Survivors

The Psychological Self

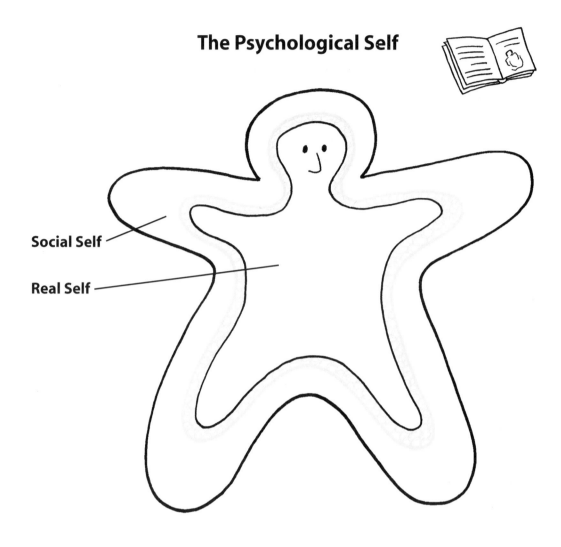

The **Social Self**, the larger, outside part of the Psychological Self, has two important jobs: communicating and protecting. It both connects you to the world and helps you feel safe in the world.

The **Real Self** has a number of special jobs and they are very different from the jobs of the Social Self:

- to make sure that the Social Self knows what feels safe and unsafe
- to create solutions to problems
- to make good decisions about actions to take
- to give permission to try new things
- to guide impulsive behavior: actions taken very quickly without planning or thinking

In order to do its work, the Real Self looks outward to the Social Self and inward to itself. One Self is not better than the other. You need both the Social Self and the Real Self to form your identity, your sense of yourself. Both affect everything you feel, think, and do. Knowing yourself means knowing from moment to moment that your Social Self and your Real Self are connected and that they need to communicate well.

When the Social Self and the Real Self don't communicate well

Two things can happen when the Social Self and the Real Self don't communicate well: uncontrolled impulsive behavior and risk-taking without awareness.

Impulsive behavior
The Real Self holds parts that are special, private and vulnerable. Like most people, you don't show your Real Self unless you feel safe. When the Social Self and the Real Self are communicating well, you take the time to see whether it's safe to show your Real Self. You look at your feelings and think about the situation before deciding to act.

When your Social Self and your Real Self aren't communicating well, you might talk about yourself and your feelings too quickly, without considering the results. You might say too much too soon to the wrong people. You might tell a new friend a secret, then find out that the friend tells the secret to others. This is called unsafe self-disclosure. It's a kind of impulsive behavior, something done on the spur of the moment, without thinking about it much or planning ahead.

Mike says...
The whole world suddenly changes. You might think that you have to sell your business or quit your job and take care of your loved one. Upon reflection, it might be better to hire a paid caregiver and remain in the position of parent/advocate. I wish I had had time to think through my first impulsive need to help.

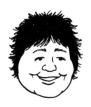

Lynne says... Understanding impulsive behavior is necessary when you care for people with brain injury. Their impulsive behavior is even more complicated than yours.

Everyone shows some impulsive behavior sometimes. However, people who have been going through a life-changing experience like brain injury often behave impulsively.

Many survivors of brain injury act impulsively in the early stages of their psychological recovery, and many caregivers do, too. One might suddenly decide to buy things he/she can't really afford. Another might suddenly decide to quit a job. What counts as impulsive behavior will be different for everyone.

The results of impulsive behavior aren't always negative, but they are often messy and hard to deal with. Most caregivers and survivors already have enough to deal with. Finding ways for the Social Self and the Real Self to communicate better will help reduce impulsive behavior and its results.

Risk-taking without awareness

When your Social Self is communicating well with the outside world and with your Real Self, you feel safe. You may take risks, but you *decide* to take them, you are *aware* of them.

When your Social Self is not communicating well with your real Self, you might feel, think, or do things that create emotional upheaval for yourself and others. This is called psychological risk, and it's the kind of risk that happens without awareness. You don't decide to do it, and you might not be aware of it. Here are some examples of feelings, thoughts and actions that result in psychological risk:

Chapter 1: Looking at the Psychological Self
When the Social Self and the Real Self don't communicate well

- You're attending a meeting with several other people. You knock over a glass of water and it spills all over some important papers. Immediately, you *feel* out of control. You *think* that you are a klutz, a failure. You *act* by making a joke about glasses that tip easily. You feel uncomfortable for the rest of the meeting but let no one know (or, you think no one knows). You spend the next few days wondering how others think about you.

- A friend tells you that you made a mistake. Immediately, you *feel* threatened. You *think* that you have to defend yourself. You *act* by shouting at the friend. Your friend says not to call any more, until you feel better.

- A driver cuts in front of you in traffic. Immediately, you *feel* angry. You *think* that the person needs to be shown a lesson. You *act* by following the car as closely as possible and blowing your car's horn over and over. The driver speeds up to get away from you and goes through a red light.

Not everything that is faced can be changed, but nothing can be changed until it is faced.

JAMES BALDWIN

Finding ways for the Social Self and the Real Self to communicate better helps reduce psychological risk. This first chapter has introduced you to the idea of the Psychological Self. Both you and the survivor need to understand this idea and the different jobs of the Social Self and the Real Self before you can expect growth and change.

The next chapter looks at the main reasons why the Social Self and the Real Self stop communicating well and helps you find ways for them to communicate better. Before looking at ways to have inner conversations, make sure that

The best bridge between hope and despair is often a good night's sleep.

ANONYMOUS

you understand the concept of the Psychological Self. Now is a good time to pause and do the two worksheets on the following pages:

- (1-2) My Psychological Self Quiz
- (1-3) Confirm Your Understanding of the Psychological Self

Helping Your Survivor

Explaining the Social Self and the Real Self to a Survivor

When you start to explain the Social Self and the Real Self to your loved one, you can use three things to help you:

1. the word explanations in this chapter
2. the picture showing the Social Self and the Real Self and their jobs
3. a large and small teddy bear, or a kangaroo with her baby in her pouch

In the Pocket Guide you will find a picture of the Social Self and the Real Self together with a word explanation.

Chapter 1: Looking at the Psychological Self
When the Social Self and the Real Self don't communicate well

Helping Your Survivor

About the teddy bear

Create a T-shirt for the teddy bear with a pouch or large pocket at the back. In the pouch, place a matching mini-bear.

Have the larger bear wear a formal black bow tie. The large bear represents the Social Self.

Make the point that different people show themselves to the world in different ways. Some people look casual (represented by the T-shirt). Some look formal (represented by the bow tie). How they look will affect how they communicate with others and how others communicate with them.

The small bear represents the Real Self. When it's hidden safe inside the Social Self, people can't see it. When it's taken out of the pouch, people can see it. Talk with your loved one about how the smaller bear might feel when inside and safe. Then talk about how the smaller bear might feel when outside and perhaps not so safe.

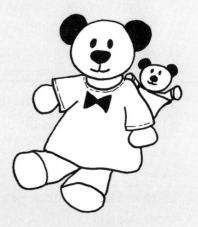

As an alternative, you could use a kangaroo with a tiny kangaroo inside her pouch.

After Brain Injury: Tools for Living
A Step-by-Step Guide for Caregivers and Survivors

W 1–2

My Psychological Self Quiz

1. Imagine being in a social situation with strangers. You are alone, perhaps anxious. Your feelings of curiosity and pleasure are absent.

2. How would you act to protect yourself from feeling too much anxiety? *(Check one.)*

   ❏ become the party clown
   ❏ retreat to the yard outside where it is quiet
   ❏ take a deep breath, count to 5, and try to look interested

3. Whichever one you picked, decide if that behavior is an expression of   *(Check one.)*

   ❏ your Social Self (whose job is to protect and communicate) OR
   ❏ your Real Self (whose jobs are to hold vulnerability, create and grow)

4. Decide which of the following are expressions of your Real Self (RS) and which are expressions of your Social Self (SS):

Expressions:	Part of my Social Self	Part of my Real Self
feeling a feeling	_____	_____
expressing a feeling	_____	_____
making an honest statement	_____	_____
wearing a mask	_____	_____
sharing a concern	_____	_____

   There are no right or wrong answers. What you will find is that the more you think about it, the more both parts of your Psychological Self are involved in many of your actions and feelings.

W 1-3   Chapter 1: Looking at the Psychological Self
When the Social Self and the Real Self don't communicate well

Confirm Your Understanding of the Psychological Self Worksheet

Part A

To have any conversation other than chit-chat, it helps to have a meaningful topic. Since we are talking about the Psychological Self, think of the most recent time you felt uncomfortable, just a little bit anxious. This will be the topic of conversation for your inner conversation.

Write a short description of what happened.
_____
_____
_____
_____
_____

How did you feel? Name the feelings.
_____   _____
_____   _____
_____   _____
_____   _____

What thoughts did you have at the time?
_____
_____
_____
_____

What did you do and how did you express yourself?
_____
_____
_____
_____

After Brain Injury: Tools for Living
A Step-by-Step Guide for Caregivers and Survivors

W 1–3

Confirm Your Understanding of the Psychological Self Worksheet

Part B

Look at the Real Self/Social Self picture below and the information you wrote on the previous page. Decide whether each bit of information is a part of your Social Self talking or a part of your Real Self talking. Write each thought, feeling, action, need, desire, or impulse in the part of this drawing where you think it belongs.

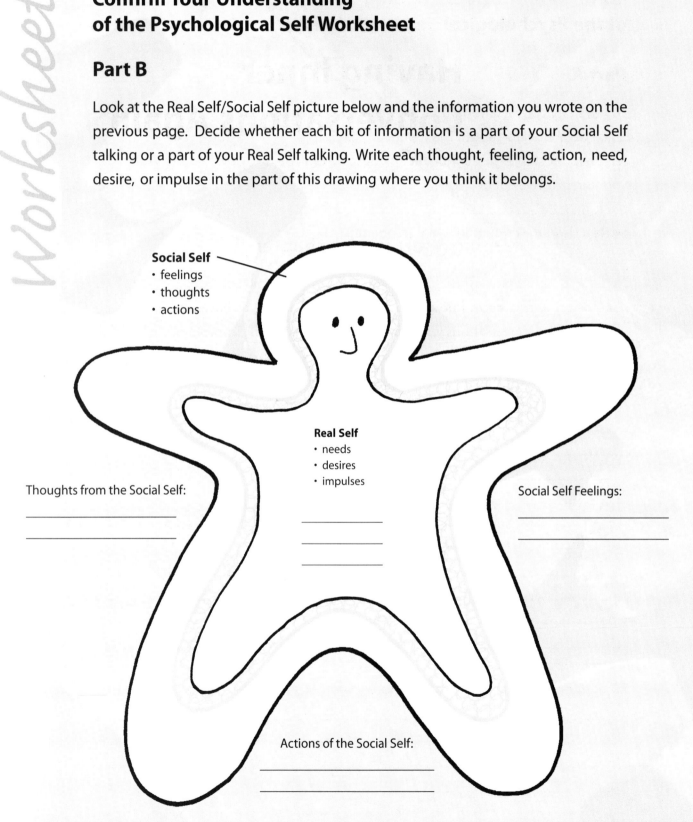

2 Having Inner Conversations Again

Learning goals for this chapter

This chapter focuses on the second important step in getting to know yourself again — learning to have inner conversations with the Psychological Self. The information here will help you in your recovery and give you ways to help your loved one.

In this chapter you will have the chance to:

- learn how to have conversations with your Psychological Self
- start to practice having conversations with your Psychological Self
- understand denial, a main stopper to conversations with your Psychological Self
- gather tools to change your conversations with your Psychological Self

Introduction

Why is it important to start having inner conversations again?

Motivation determines what you do. Attitude determines how well you do it. Action determines the outcome.

ANONYMOUS

Chapter 1 talked about an important first step in getting to know yourself again — looking at the Psychological Self, the part of you in charge of psychological recovery. In the upheaval and loss after brain injury, the Psychological Self can get out of balance. The Social Self may be so strong that it keeps you from reaching your Real Self. The Real Self may be so well hidden that it seems no one is home. Or the Real Self may be so strong that it seems the Social Self has run away. Chapter 1 showed some of the things that can happen when the Psychological Self is out of balance and the Social Self and the Real Self don't communicate well.

Recovering psychologically after brain injury has been called "the self learning to have a conversation with itself." In other words, recovering psychologically means helping the Social Self and the Real Self learn to communicate better with each other. When the Social Self and the Real Self start communicating, you will be able to have inner conversations and start knowing yourself again. That's the focus of this chapter.

When are you ready to have inner conversations again?

As a caregiver, you know you are on your way to having these important inner conversations when you are:

- showing an attitude of willingness

- contacting your Social Self and your Real Self

- understanding denial as a stopper to inner conversations

Willpower and willingness

In the first stage of recovery, the physical stage, you probably called on your willpower over and over again. Your loved one did, too. Willpower is the part of your Real Self that drives you to get something done, no matter what. It combines such things as hard work, determination, and courage, and helps people achieve amazing goals.

Willpower worked very well to get you and your loved one through this first stage of physical recovery. You know what it took for you to stay by the side of your loved one as she/he did whatever it took to regain physical strength and skills. You know what it took for your loved one to regain the physical abilities he/she has now. You can both be proud of your success.

Willingness is absolutely essential for change to happen.

Helping Your Survivor

The Chinese Finger Toy

A child's toy from China can help survivors of brain injury understand the difference between willpower and willingness. This toy shows that sometimes all the willpower in the world can't bring about change, and only willingness will work.

For many years, people in China have made a child's toy called a finger puzzle or finger trap. The original puzzles were cylinders made of tightly woven bamboo. Now they're made of woven plastic and are sold around the world. The cylinders are only large enough to fit on the end of a finger or thumb.

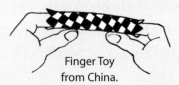

Finger Toy from China.

To use the puzzle, put one finger from each hand into the cylinder. (You could use your thumbs instead.) After you insert your fingers in the ends of the puzzle, try to pull your fingers out.

Like most people, you will probably try to pull your fingers out with brute force. This is an example of willpower at work. However, pulling only makes the cylinder grip your fingers more tightly. Willpower does not solve the problem. In fact, willpower makes the problem worse.

Think about other ways to solve the puzzle. Let go of any frustration and stay open to new ideas.

You will discover that the only way you can remove your fingers from the puzzle is by relaxing, then gently pushing in and twisting. That way the puzzle loosens its grip enough to let your fingers go. This is an example of creative thinking, of willingness to try something different, and it solves the problem.

After you learn this for yourself, you can use this tool to teach your loved one the same important concept.

Chapter 2: Having Inner Conversations Again
Showing an Attitude of Willingness

Now that you and your loved one have entered the stage of psychological recovery, you may find that both of you have over-learned how to use your willpower. You're so used to using your willpower that you've forgotten there are other ways to bring about change.

You've probably noticed by now that willpower works very well to bring about physical change, but it doesn't work very well to bring about psychological change. What's needed for this kind of change is willingness.

Willingness is being ready to take a risk and learn something new. Willingness allows you to be curious, open, and exploring even when you feel scared or frustrated. Willingness is absolutely essential. It prepares the way for the changes that allow inner conversations to start again.

In recovery, sometimes you might find it hard to know when you need willpower and when you need willingness. Like most people, when change is needed, you will probably try willpower first. If the change you want does not come about, then try using willingness. Usually you will find that being open to new learning puts you on the path to psychological recovery.

Both willpower and willingness require courage and commitment of the Psychological Self. Both also require strength. Willpower requires physical strength and commitment to personal goals. Willingness requires the emotional strength to face the feelings that come when risking new healing and growth. That makes willingness very important in helping the Social Self and the Real Self start communicating again.

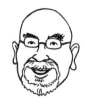

**Mike says …
The Chinese Finger Toy reminds us that pulling against each other doesn't work. Working together to find solutions does work.**

Consider how hard it is to change yourself, and you will understand what little chance you have trying to change others.

ANONYMOUS

Here's how willingness helps you start having inner conversations between your Social Self and your Real Self. If you have willingness, you are willing to:

- learn more about yourself

- try new things

- continue even though you feel uncomfortable, confused, or frustrated

Without this attitude of willingness, having inner conversations will not happen. That is the power of willingness. If you allow yourself to listen to your Psychological Self — to hear the conversation between your Social Self and your Real Self — gradually you will begin to know just what you need to hear in order to heal and grow.

Helping Your Survivor

Willpower and Willingness

The strength in willpower lies in the courage, determination, and strength to keep on building physical skills and abilities.

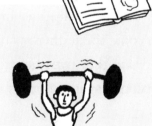

The strength in willingness lies in the courage and commitment to stay open to learning new things, even when they make you feel anxious.

Chapter 2: Having Inner Conversations Again
Showing an Attitude of Willingness

What's the first step in allowing this inner conversation to happen? Be willing to put aside all your questions about whether learning how to have inner conversations will work for your loved one. Start working on your own inner conversations. There may be bumps as you learn how to know yourself again. By staying open and willing, you will find that you can contact your Social Self and your Real Self and start hearing them clearly within you.

Giving inner conversations a chance

Most people need more than willingness to have inner conversations. They also need to take some action. Here is one way of making sure your inner conversations have a chance to happen:

- Set aside some time just for yourself. Maybe start with five minutes a day. Later you can try to increase this time to 10 minutes or more.

- Find a place on your own where you can focus and where you won't be interrupted.

- Sit rather than lie down. You want to have an inner conversation, not a nap.

- Before you start, set an egg timer to keep track of the time you want to spend. That way you won't distract yourself by looking at your watch or peeking at the clock.

- Sit in silence. Or, if it suits you better, put on soft music that you find soothing.

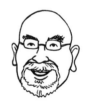

Mike says...
I found going for walks gave me the opportunity to have my inner talks.

43

- Focus inside yourself until your time is up.

- Stay willing to keep at it, even when your mind wanders and your toe itches.

The eyes of men speak words the tongue cannot pronounce.

NATIVE AMERICAN PROVERB

When you've finished, try to talk or write about what you learned during your inner conversation. Talk to someone else, speak into a tape recorder, or write in a journal.

This is a good time to start the daily habit of writing in a journal. Try to spend 10 minutes a day writing about even one detail of your inner conversation. Try to identify when your Social Self was speaking and when it was listening. Then do the same for your Real Self. If you don't have time or energy to write, try drawing pictures, then add words later. This journal is different from the one you may already be keeping about your loved one. Both are important.

Keeping a Journal

Your journal can be a small spiral-bound booklet you've bought specially, or as simple as lined paper stapled together. To remind you of the Social Self and the Real Self, try taping or gluing into the front of your journal a copy of the Psychological Self = Social Self + Real Self picture you saw in Chapter 1. Or you could draw a picture of your own.

To make it easy and simple for you to write in your journal, you could place headings like these on each page: Date, Time and Place, Topic, Social Self — thoughts and actions, and Real Self — feelings, needs, desires, and impulses. Look on the next page for a sample:

- (2-1) My Journal — A Blank Journal Page

W 2-1

Chapter 2: Having Inner Conversations Again
Showing an Attitude of Willingness

My Journal — A Blank Journal Page

Date _____ Time and Place _____

Topic _____

Social Self — thoughts and actions
_____
_____
_____
_____
_____
_____
_____
_____
_____
_____
_____
_____

Real Self — feelings, needs, desires, and impulses
_____
_____
_____
_____
_____
_____
_____
_____
_____
_____
_____
_____

Contacting your Social Self and your Real Self

Nobody can be exactly like me. Even I have trouble doing it.

Tallulah Bankhead

Having a conversation involves both a speaker and a listener. As a caregiver, you are used to talking with and listening to others. In order to have inner conversations, you need to talk with and listen to your Social Self and your Real Self. Your Social Self and your Real Self also need to talk with and listen to each other. That way you will come to understand a few things about yourself:

- how you feel (even if you feel absent or flat)

- what feels good, positive, or healing

- what feels bad, negative, or scary

- why you feel that way

- what you need to do to feel better

- what you need to do to feel safe

- what you need to do next to heal and grow

Like many people, when you first start trying to have inner conversations, you might find that your Real Self seems to have disappeared. All you hear is your Social Self chattering busily away about details and things, not about feelings. You may start to think about something you forgot to do this morning. You may start to make up a list of groceries to buy at the store. You may start to wonder whether you should do a wash this evening.

Chapter 2: Having Inner Conversations Again
Contacting your Social Self and your Real Self

Some people describe the endless chatter in their heads as the Social Self running out of control. Your Real Self, your inner self, has been buried by everything that has happened since the brain injury. One person describes the experience this way: "I can't find my Real Self. I have no feelings. I feel empty all the time. I don't even dream. I wear a mask all the time."

How can you tell for sure that your Social Self is controlling things? Slow down and listen carefully to your inner conversations. The Social Self generally speaks in longer sentences, with longer words, than the Real Self. Thinking in sentences is normally just what you do when talking with the outside world. The Real Self speaks simply. And, if the Real Self and the Social Self are truly communicating, the Social Self also speaks simply, with short sentences.

Lynne says... Relax. If you find all your inner conversations begin with paragraphs, go take a bath. Relax. Come back and try again later. Too many words are usually a sign of trying too hard.

Some people trying to have inner conversations find that the Social Self has disappeared. One person describes it this way: "I have lost my Social Self. My Real Self is 'on' 100 per cent of the time. Private feelings just pop out when I'm not expecting them. It seems like no thought is going on and that I'm not in control."

What are you saying when you talk about struggles between the Social Self and the Real Self? You are saying that you have lost your ability to have an inner conversation with your Psychological Self. The Social Self and the Real Self are operating separately instead of cooperating. They have lost the willingness and the ability to listen to each other.

The first duty of love is to listen.

T‍ILLICH

Think about the best conversations you have with a good friend, where you both end up feeling noticed, appreciated, and listened to. In these conversations, the speaker speaks and the listener listens. You then change places. The same is true for your inner conversations. You'll know when healing and growth is starting to be possible because your Social Self and your Real Self will be acting equally as listeners and speakers.

Understanding Denial as a Stopper to Inner Conversations

So far in this chapter, you may have tried some inner conversations and started a journal. You know that you can use inner conversations to contact your Social Self and your Real Self. You know that all the psychological work you're doing to make inner conversations happen is helping you start to know yourself again.

Just as important as knowing how to have inner conversations is understanding what stops them and learning how to deal with the stopper. Denial is the main stopper of inner conversations.

Chapter 2: Having Inner Conversations Again
Understanding Denial as a Stopper to Inner Conversations

Denial — the automatic protection mechanism

Your Psychological Self has taken good care of you since the brain injury happened to your loved one. Remember how scared, insecure, and helpless you felt when the brain injury first happened? Somehow you set aside most of those feelings to help you get through that awful time. You went into the type of shock that lasts for a time. This shock period helped so that you wouldn't be overwhelmed and stop doing what you needed to do — support your loved one the best you could.

After brain injury and other huge life-changing events, the Psychological Self automatically acts to protect you. This is the third part of the Psychological Self at work — the automatic protection mechanism of denial. This automatic protection mechanism acts like chain-mail armor. You needed this wonderful protection right after the brain injury happened to your loved one. It gave your Social Self extra strength to help you stay on top of all the details involved in dealing with family and friends and supporting your loved one during her/his physical recovery. It kept you from being overwhelmed with feelings. You can feel grateful that your automatic protection mechanism did such a good job then.

The problem is that the automatic protection mechanism of denial often carries on long after it's needed. It does such a good job that many caregivers and survivors become comfortable with that way of handling things. You too might find that you keep acting as though the chaos of the early days of the brain injury is still happening. You might react to everything as though it were another emergency, another traumatic event. You might just feel empty inside. You might have forgotten that life wasn't always this way.

If you are willing to admit you are wrong when you are wrong, you are all right.

ANONYMOUS

This is another way inner conversations can help. By helping your Social Self and your Real Self communicate better, you can reassure the part of yourself still reacting automatically. "The worst of the brain injury is over," says your Social Self. Your Real Self says: "No, that is not true." Denial protects you from feeling this struggle too much. The truth is, whatever happens next, feelings and inner conversations that comfort you are possible.

With that reassurance, you can start letting go of your automatic protection mechanism of denial gradually and safely. You can start honoring the needs of your Real Self and allowing your feelings to show. Sometimes you will still need to use more of your Social Self to connect with others safely. By listening, you will find out which part of your Psychological Self needs expression at any one moment.

Mike says...
I remember giving my first speech. I felt uncomfortable, insecure, thinking I'd look foolish, make mistakes. I stood at the podium, shaking inside. It went well, but inside, I was still talking to my Real Self about failure.

Negative, judgmental self-talk

Especially while you are trying to let go of your automatic protection mechanism, how you listen to your Psychological Self is very important.

Think about a time when someone said something that stopped you from trying something. How did you feel? Did you keep listening to yourself and what you really wanted to do? Did you get angry? Did you give up the idea? When you remember how you felt, you'll know that opinions and negative judgment are powerful stoppers even without life-changing events like brain injury.

Like many people, you might have learned how to listen, but only critically, with opinions. You might not need someone else to give you negative opinions and judgments.

Chapter 2: Having Inner Conversations Again
Understanding Denial as a Stopper to Inner Conversations

You might do that all on your own with negative, judgmental self-talk. Negative, judgmental self-talk happens when you tell yourself that something you've done or something you want to do is bad, stupid, wrong, ridiculous, too much, not enough, or too risky.

Now that you're starting to have inner conversations and paying attention to them, you're probably noticing your negative, judgmental self-talk more. You know what a stopper such self-talk can be.

"Why would you want to do that?"

"You're doing it that way?"

"That's never worked before."

For many people, negative, judgmental self-talk becomes a habit, something they do often without thinking much about it. If you have this habit, maybe you developed it after your loved one had a brain injury. Or you might have talked this way to your Psychological Self for a long time before.

Like all habits, this one can be changed with willingness. Being willing to try is the all-important first step. Give yourself permission to live without judgment. Next time you try to have an inner conversation, pause and ask yourself, "What does my Real Self want?" Then listen for the answer. At first, you may hear negative, judgmental self-talk. Or you may hear just silence. Respect this. Respect that your Real Self cannot quite join the conversation yet.

Then try asking yourself: "What can I do to feel more safe, in just this moment?" Listen. If your Real Self is still silent, remember that your Social Self can communicate with your Real Self. Ask your Social Self to help. Your Social Self could answer questions like these:

- Do I need a quieter space?

- Would some quiet music help me?

- Do I have an hour a week or 15 minutes a day set aside just for me?

- Do I need to be alone and just relax?

- Do I need to talk with someone?

What can I do to feel more safe, in just this moment?

You might remain in this speaking, questioning stage for minutes, days, or weeks. You may not be able to hear your Real Self. It may take time for you to hear, truly hear, the Real Self's answer about what you need to feel safe. Don't give up. Remain willing to learn something new about yourself. That is what's required.

What happens if weeks go by, and you still hear either negative, judgmental self-talk or silence? Then it might help to make a commitment like this: "I promise myself that each time I hear a negative judgment or criticism of myself I am going to say STOP, and LET IT GO. I'm not going to examine it. I'm just going to let it go." You might have so many negatives inside you that your Real Self is doing exactly what it needs to do. It is hiding until it feels safe.

Practice this commitment for a week. You might find that you have reduced your negative, judgmental self-talk or even got rid of it altogether. You might still hear just silence from your Real Self. Keep listening with patience and willingness. If you still hear only silence, perhaps look at it this way: The silence is a message. At a deeper level, maybe something else is happening. Maybe you are still being protected from all your fears and worries. Maybe it's time to take a closer look at denial.

Denial is the main automatic stopper of inner conversation, and it's a very powerful one. Denial results from the Psychological Self's automatic reaction to two things:

- physical effects of brain injury or other major trauma

- psychological effects from the loss and upheaval resulting from brain injury or other major trauma

Dealing with the survivor's brain-based denial
Helping professionals notice that in the early stages of physical recovery, many survivors of brain injury have a special type of denial or lack of awareness. It is called physical or brain-based denial, and it is very different from psychological denial.

Three kinds of physically based types of denial are very common in survivors in the early stages of recovery, before damaged brain tissues have had a chance to heal: perseveration, confabulation, and inability to focus on the Psychological Self.

Consciousness: that annoying time between naps.

ANONYMOUS

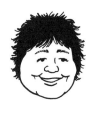

Lynne says... These denial behaviors have one thing in common: They are not part of the Psychological Self that we have been talking about. Rather, they are part of physical healing. However, these behaviors are often tiring for caregivers to be around, especially when caregivers are dealing with their own healing. That's why we are inserting them here.

Here is a brief description of these physically based types of denial, along with some suggestions about how you as a caregiver can handle them.

Perseveration

The survivor showing perseveration says or does the same things over and over again. Most caregivers find this behavior tiring to be around. As you probably know by now, trying to stop or interrupt your loved one doesn't often work. Even when it does work, it doesn't work for long. However, you or someone else can usually distract your loved one long enough for you to have a short break from listening to or watching the behavior.

Do not expect an intervention to heal this behavior. For most survivors, over time, healing of the tissues gradually heals perseveration. The best treatment for you and your loved one? Ignore the behavior. Find other people to "spot" you for relief. Know that this, too, will probably pass.

"Can we go out now?"

"Are we leaving soon?"

"When are we going out?"

"Let's go. When are we going?"

"Are we leaving soon?"

Confabulation

Confabulation happens when the survivor replaces fact with fantasy. Brains are designed to make thoughts and stories flow and make sense. After brain injury, the survivor's brain tries to fill in the blanks where facts are missing from memories. Once the survivor creates these confabulated memories, they feel real to the survivor even though they did not happen as the survivor remembers them. This seems to be an automatic, not consciously thought-out, behavior that is not open to change.

To you and others, this form of denial looks and sounds as though your loved one is lying. However, lying usually happens consciously, with the liar knowing that she/he is lying. Confabulation is also not story-telling. Story-telling happens when someone tells a story and the storyteller and the listeners know that the facts are made up. You may find yourself needing to explain the difference between story-telling and confabulation to family and friends.

The best treatment for you and the survivor? Allow time to do its magic. Know that this behavior too will probably fade. Don't take the behavior personally. Let family and friends know that it's normal for survivors to confabulate in various stages of recovery. Some recover, and some carry this with them.

Inability to focus on the Psychological Self

Early in their physical recovery, people with brain injuries cannot focus their attention for long. Sometimes their attention span may be as little as a few seconds or minutes. This is different from forgetting, and it doesn't mean that

**Mike says . . .
I used to think confabulation was deliberate story-telling and lying. Now, after time, I realize it felt real true to the person, but didn't happen. I spent a lot of time trying to convince someone who couldn't hear what I was saying.**

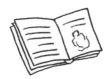

Anyone who thinks that they are too small to make a difference, has never been in bed with a mosquito.

Anonymous

your loved one isn't listening to you and others. At this stage, most survivors do not show much interest in or anxiety about the Psychological Self. You may want your loved one to start on psychological recovery. You may want to talk with your loved one about the Social Self and the Real Self and inner conversations. But it's too soon.

As with confabulation and perseveration, you will find that over time, your loved one will start to focus for longer periods. Gradually, most survivors will reach the place where they can focus enough to start working on psychological recovery. What can help you, the caregiver, during this time? Try to be patient. Remember that your loved one's inability to focus is not intentional, but the result of brain injury.

These physically based denial behaviors can be very frustrating for you as a caregiver and for others dealing with your loved one. Now is a good time to pause and do the worksheet on the following pages:

- (2-2) SST (Stop, Still Myself and Think) Instructional Aid

Even though the SST focuses on treating impulsive anger outbursts, you can adapt the SST to help you reduce your frustration as you spend time with your loved one when he/she is using denial behaviors.

SST (Stop-Still-Think) Instructional Aid

After brain injury, thoughts, feelings, and actions can "jump out" without any planning. A person with a brain injury might have a "short fuse" or get angry too quickly or too much for a given situation. This is not a behavioral or an emotional problem. It is the result of disordered impulses. The person with a brain injury needs to re-learn how to control impulses.

Stop-Still-Think (SST) is a method for helping your loved one interrupt impulses, whether they are feelings, thoughts, or actions. The SST Aid consists of two sizes of cue cards.

SST stands for Stop, Still, Think.

Your goal is to use the SST aid to help your loved one train herself/himself to think of Stop-Still-Think every time she/he faces a situation needing help with impulse control. Both the large and small sets act as reminders to your loved one to stop, take a few breaths, and think before taking action. You can also use this tool for yourself.

Example of a Small SST Cue Card

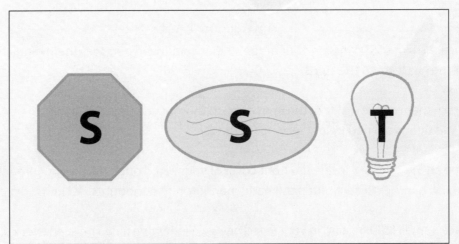

After Brain Injury: Tools for Living
A Step-by-Step Guide for Caregivers and Survivors

More About SST

As soon as you feel a twinge of a feeling or the beginning of a reactionary thought (a thought in reaction to another person's actions which affect you), follow the steps below.

 First, just for the moment, stop everything you are doing. If you are walking, STOP. If you are talking, STOP.

 Next, take some deep breaths. For just a few moments, focus only on this calming breathing. Use the wavy line to remind you of this inner calmness. Breathe your way there.

 Then, having stilled yourself, take another moment and ask yourself the following question: "Is there something I think or feel needs to be done now or should I hold my reaction inside me?"

SST can be used as a method for teaching systematic thinking to overcome impulsive thinking. SST replaces the Think-Do way of taking action impulsively with three steps — Stop, Still, Think — that happen before any action is taken. Placed in the wallet and throughout the home or at work, SST cue cards act as constant reminders of the three SST steps.

You will find a set of SST cue cards inserted into this book. The SST cue cards can be used in these ways:

- Place the large SST cards on your fridge so that your loved one sees them regularly until she/he has learned the steps.

- Attach them on the inside of the front door, to prompt your loved one to gather together all the things needed before leaving for the day.

- Tape an SST cue card inside the front cover of your loved one's daytimer or organizer, to remind him/her to carry out systematic, non-impulsive thoughts, feelings, or actions.

- Place a small SST cue card in your loved one's wallet where it can be seen every time the wallet is opened.

Chapter 2: Having Inner Conversations Again
Understanding Denial as a Stopper to Inner Conversations

Dealing with your own self-based denial

Everyone needs ways to protect themselves from too much anxiety. As mentioned earlier in this chapter, denial helps people cope with huge amounts of stress and anxiety after sudden, life-changing events. Denial helped protect you as a caregiver in the time after your loved one experienced brain injury, and denial continues to protect you now. As an automatic protection mechanism, denial gave your Social Self extra strength to help you stay on top of all the details involved in dealing with family and friends and supporting your loved one during physical recovery. It helped keep you from being overwhelmed with feelings.

Denial is the way your Psychological Self protects you when you have too much upheaval, loss, and worry in your Real Self. Denial helps you set aside your feelings and do what you need to do. This kind of denial is often called self-based denial because it comes from your Psychological Self. Self-based denial can be described this way:

- It's used by everyone now and then.

- It's a normal, healthy response to feeling too much upheaval, loss, or worry.

- It automatically happens, with no thought, planning or awareness required from you.

- It helps you behave in a socially acceptable way while it protects you from feeling too much anxiety.

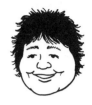

Lynne says...
Many psychologists and psychoanalysts have spent their careers observing and studying the forms of protection that I refer to as self-based denial. Sigmund Freud, the founder of psychoanalysis, called these forms of denial 'defence mechanisms' because their purpose was to defend, or protect, the Self. Other terms for self-based denial: psychogenic denial or psychologically based denial.

There are many kinds of self-based denial. Here are some shown by many caregivers, survivors, and other people with too much upheaval, loss, or worry in their lives:

- **Humor.** You use humor to distract yourself and others from an uncomfortable situation. For example, if you feel uncomfortable in medical places, you might constantly make jokes while in a hospital. Joking allows you to stay in a situation that's uncomfortable and protects you from feeling too much anxiety.

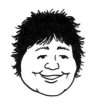

**Lynne says...
People with brain injuries also have psychogenic, or self-based, denial. It is just that early on, they also have the brain-based kind.**

- **Regression.** You go back to a less adult way of behaving, such as stamping your feet or throwing things.

- **Not knowing.** When asked, you do not seem to know what you're feeling, thinking, or doing in the moment. Someone asks, "How are you?" and you answer, "I don't know." If the person tries to force you to answer, you might feel overwhelmed by all your worries and fears.

- **Intellectualization.** You use ideas and words to build a wall between you and your feelings. You talk only about ideas and words, not about feelings you might be having.

- **Projection.** You blame others for your shortcomings. For example, you blame others for "making" you angry. You don't place responsibility for your anger where it belongs ...with you.

Chapter 2: Having Inner Conversations Again
Understanding Denial as a Stopper to Inner Conversations

- **Rationalization.** You try to explain your behavior with reasons that sound true, but aren't. For example, you arrive late for a meeting and say that the traffic slowed you down, when in fact you left home too late to allow for traffic slow-downs.

- **Reaction formation.** You act opposite to the expected, and usually you react with rage. For example, when hammering in a nail, you hit your thumb. Instead of showing that you're hurt, you angrily throw the hammer away.

Stress is when you wake up screaming and you realize you haven't fallen asleep yet.

ANONYMOUS

As these examples show, everyone uses self-based denial now and then. It's normal. It's the automatic protection mechanism at work. Self-based denial only becomes a problem when it's used so much that it stops inner conversations and slows down psychological recovery. The next and final section of this chapter talks about how to make your inner conversations safe so that you can start getting to know yourself again.

Before looking at ways to make inner conversations safe, now is a good time to pause and do the worksheet on the following pages:

- (2-3) Exploring My Self-Based Denial

After Brain Injury: Tools for Living
A Step-by-Step Guide for Caregivers and Survivors

W 2-3

Exploring My Self-Based Denial Worksheet

Getting to know yourself again means looking at some of the ways in which you have protected yourself from loss, worry, and upheaval. Think of times when you used the kinds of denial shown in the chart below. Use the blank space to write a bit about your behavior. What caused it? What happened next? Another question you could ask yourself: "Do I still use this kind of denial often?"

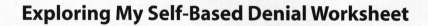

Kinds of Self-Based Denial	Description
Regression	Reverting to an earlier, less adult way of acting (for example, stamping feet when angry).
Your personal example:	_____
Wit & Humor	Using puns and other humor to distract yourself and others from uncomfortable feelings (for example, you act as the jokester, class clown, or party animal).
Your personal example:	_____
Intellectualization	You use ideas and words to build a wall between you and your feelings. You talk only about ideas and words, not about feelings you might be having.
Your personal example:	_____

Chapter 2: Having Inner Conversations Again
Understanding Denial as a Stopper to Inner Conversations

Not Knowing   When asked, you don't seem to know what you're feeling, thinking, or doing in the moment. Someone asks, "How are you?" and you answer, "I don't know." If the person tries to force you to answer, you immediately feel overwhelmed by all your worries and fears.

Your personal example: _____
_____
_____

Rationalization   You try to explain your behavior with reasons that sound true, but aren't. For example, you arrive late for a meeting and say that the traffic slowed you down, when in fact you left home too late to allow for traffic slow-downs.

Your personal example: _____
_____
_____

Projection   You blame others for your shortcomings. For example, you blame others for "making" you angry. You don't place responsibility for your anger where it belongs — with you.

Your personal example: _____
_____
_____

Reaction Formation   You act opposite to the expected and usually you react with rage. For example, when hammering in a nail, you hit your thumb. You throw the hammer away angrily.

Your personal example: _____
_____
_____

Helping Your Survivor

Self-Based Denial

Remember the picture of the Psychological Self, showing the outer Social Self and the inner Real Self? Denial is like a suit of armor protecting the Real Self. This armor protects the Real Self when it's filled with upheaval, loss, or worry after brain injury.

This armor gives your Real Self a container for all the anxiety you feel. It helps you set aside your feelings and do what you need to do. Humor is an example of how self-based denial works:

- Something happens in the outside world or inside you. Perhaps someone says to you, "You're lazy. You should do more."

- When you hear the remark, you feel very upset, worried, angry, and afraid. Your inner self, your Real Self, is immediately overwhelmed with feelings.

- The armor between the Social Self and the Real Self automatically acts to protect your Real Self and keep all your feelings inside.

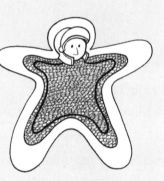

- You make a joke. You say, "I'll order another pair of legs today."

- Everyone around you laughs.

- While you're all laughing, and for a time afterward, what the person said feels less upsetting, worrying, and scary. The joke has helped you get through an uncomfortable time.

Can you think of ways you have used humor to help you through times when you felt upset, worried, angry, or afraid?

After you've introduced humor and talked about some examples, you can introduce the other kinds of self-based denial: regression, not knowing, intellectualization, projection, rationalization, and reaction formation.

Making inner conversations safe

Now that you have read this chapter, you might be starting to realize that denial and negative, judgmental self-talk often stop inner conversations between your Social Self and your Real Self. If you truly want to start to recover psychologically and have inner conversations, it's time to recognize that you need emotional safety for growth. Then it's time to make a few commitments:

- looking at how denial serves you

- stopping negative, judgmental self-talk

- creating the safety it takes to start having inner conversations

Looking at how denial serves you

In earlier sections of this chapter, you saw how self-based denial served you well when you felt upset, worried, or afraid. You might ask, "If denial is the body's built-in method of self-protection, shouldn't I just leave it be?"

Safety comes first.

Safety is absolutely necessary for growth to happen.

The short answer is yes. Safety comes first. Safety is absolutely necessary for growth to happen. You must feel safe inside and outside before you can start to let go of self-based denial. You must feel safe inside and outside before you can start to let go of the stoppers to your inner conversations.

The long answer is that by paying attention to what you need to feel safe, you are preparing yourself for change. You are opening the way to having healing conversations between your Social Self and your Real Self. You are starting on a path of healing and growth that will help you get to know yourself again. The same is true for the survivor you care for and about.

Stopping negative, judgmental self-talk

As you read earlier in this chapter, negative, judgmental self-talk happens when you tell yourself that something you've done or something you want to do is bad, stupid, wrong, ridiculous, too much, not enough, or too risky. You may tell yourself things like this: "Shape up" or "Get serious" or "Try harder" or "Stop feeling."

**Mike says . . .
It is important to be positive with your loved one, but it is even more important to be positive with yourself. It helps you to start crawling out of the dark hole of despair.**

Negative, judgmental self-talk does make you feel safe for a while. It stops you from doing anything risky that might make you uncomfortable. But it's not behavior that will let you heal and grow. It stops your Real Self from being heard. Sometimes the way to stop negative, judgmental self-talk is to practice positive self-talk. Here are some ideas:

- Pay attention to the feelings you have and the actions you take when you don't feel safe. For example, you might say, "I must be reacting to some inside worry, because I just started blaming someone else again."

- Tell yourself when you feel unsafe. For example, say, "I don't feel safe saying this. It doesn't matter why right now, but I don't feel safe." Then don't say what you were about to say.

- Be your own best friend. Comfort yourself, and give yourself pep talks. For example, say, "It's okay that I said that. It could have been worse. Good for me!"

Doing what it takes to start having inner conversations

Right now, it might be enough for you to just get through the day or the moment. This is daily survival mode in terms of psychological recovery. That's where you need to be, so just accept that for now. In this stage, you have probably started to notice that you are using self-based denial and other ways to protect yourself, to help you feel safe and do what you have to do.

But if you have been reading this chapter, you have been reaching out for ways to heal and grow psychologically. You want to start having inner conversations and getting to know yourself again. You know that in order to start on that path, your Real Self needs to feel safe.

Think back to the sections of this chapter that talked about ways of stopping negative, judgmental self-talk and making inner conversations possible. That information can be summarized this way, with one important addition at the end:

- Next time you try to have an inner conversation, pause and ask yourself, "What does my Real Self need?" Then listen for the answer. At first, you may hear negative, judgmental self-talk. Or you may hear just silence. Respect this. Respect that your Real Self cannot quite join the conversation yet.

- Then try asking yourself: "What can I do to feel more safe, in just this moment?" Listen. If your Real Self is still silent, remember that your Social Self can communicate with your Real Self. Ask your Social Self to help.

> Right now, it might be enough for you to just get through the day or the moment.

- If you still hear only silence, make yourself this promise: "I promise myself that each time I hear a negative judgment or criticism of myself I am going to say STOP, and LET IT GO. I'm not going to examine it. I'm just going to let it go."

- If you still hear only silence, perhaps look at it this way: The silence is a message. At a deeper level, something else is happening. Maybe you are still being protected from all your fears and worries. Maybe it's time to look at self-based denial.

- Here's the addition: If letting go of negative, judgmental self-talk doesn't work and you've spent weeks patiently listening, maybe you need help unsticking the stopper to your inner conversations. Maybe your automatic protective mechanism is working overtime. Maybe you're stuck in some self-based denial behaviors. You probably need to increase your sense of inner safety.

This might be a good time to seek out someone qualified to act in the role of listener for you.

This might be a good time to seek out someone qualified to act in the role of listener for you. Counsellors and psychotherapists have spent years learning how to help others build their internal safety and get to know themselves again. Let them help you.

Once you are well on the way to having inner conversations and getting to know yourself again, you can continue to heal by starting to work on your emotional recovery. That's the topic of the next chapter.

3 Recovering Emotionally

Learning goals for this chapter

This chapter looks at emotional recovery in several ways. First, to help you understand why you feel the way you do, the chapter shows the experiences that many other caregivers like you have gone through. Next the chapter helps you identify the feelings you're having now. Finally, the chapter shows you that there is light at the end of the tunnel. You *can* look forward to the time when you have energy for other things.

In this chapter, you will have a chance to:

- look at core issues in emotional recovery
- explore five stages in emotional recovery and healing
- come to understand your own core issues
- find practical tools for guiding your recovery
- identify trauma roles and think about ways of changing them
- learn how to help the survivor in her/his emotional recovery

Introduction

A person is grown up not when they can take care of themselves, but when they can take care of others.

ANONYMOUS

Chapters 1 and 2 looked at the first step that you, the caregiver, could take to start recovering psychologically after your loved one started to recover physically from brain injury. This first step, getting to know yourself again, involves understanding the Psychological Self and how it works. Chapter 1 introduced you to the main parts of the Psychological Self — the outer Social Self, the inner Real Self, and the automatic protection mechanism of denial.

In order for you to start getting to know yourself again, the Social Self and the Real Self must start communicating well and allowing you to have inner conversations. Chapter 2 showed you how to start having these inner conversations again. It also gave you some ideas about how to deal with denial, the automatic protection mechanism that is the main stopper to these inner conversations.

Chapter 3 helps you continue the healing and growth you started in Chapters 1 and 2. You've read those chapters and used the worksheets and other resources. You're starting to have inner conversations and you're getting to know yourself again. Now you are ready to start recovering emotionally from the loss and upheaval you experienced after the brain injury happened.

Chapter 3: Recovering Emotionally
Introduction

What does it mean to recover emotionally?

Like most caregivers at this stage of recovery, you might find that you have quite a mix of feelings. That's normal for people after they've had huge upheavals in their lives.

On the positive side, you know that the survivor has come a long way, and you feel happy and relieved about that. There's so much to celebrate. You look forward to watching the survivor continue to heal and grow, and you look forward to being part of that healing and growth.

But you might have other feelings that aren't so positive — loss, sadness, anger, confusion, numbness, and worry. These feelings might be shutting you down and making it hard for you to connect with others at a time when you really need support. You might feel that your feelings are running the show and that you're spending too much of your energy trying to manage them. Recovering emotionally means bringing back balance to your feelings, so that they're part of you but don't control you.

Emotional recovery also means allowing growth. Allowing yourself to grow and change is a very important part of recovering emotionally. It means opening up before you know what comes next in the process of recovery. It involves risk, too, but you get to control how much risk you want to take and when you will take it.

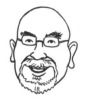

Mike says . . . Recovering emotionally is something I find so important. You need to take care of yourself first. You can't be a basket case and help someone else!

Why is it important to recover emotionally?

Humans are like tea bags. They never realize their strength until they are put in hot water.

ANONYMOUS

Getting back the ability to look inside yourself and become more aware of yourself is an important step toward recovering psychologically from trauma like brain injury. Another important step is to use this ability as you bring back balance to your feelings.

Why is that important? Think back to the last time you felt very, very tired. Put yourself back in that moment. Why do you feel so tired? You could have a physical reason. Maybe you stayed up all night caring for your loved one. Maybe you have the flu. Maybe your back hurts. It might take most of your energy just to get through the day.

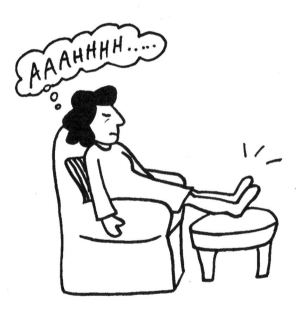

You could have an emotional reason for feeling so tired. Maybe you feel worried about money. Maybe you're feeling depressed. Maybe you're finding it hard to focus on anything. The result is the same, whether the reason is physical or emotional. It takes most of your energy just to get through the day.

Chapter 3: Recovering Emotionally
Introduction

That's why recovering emotionally is important. Not dealing with your feelings takes a lot of energy. Until you start recovering emotionally, you might continue to spend most of your energy just getting through the day. You might find your thoughts and actions affected in ways that are hard for you to deal with. You won't have the energy to heal and grow.

What is trauma?

Since your loved one survived brain injury, you've probably heard the word "trauma" often from healthcare providers. Trauma describes any event that does the following three things:

- happens suddenly, without warning

- brings about catastrophic change and loss that is soul-shattering and life-changing

- usually takes a long time to heal

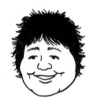

An earthquake that takes place in a populated area is one example of an event that brings trauma. An earthquake happens suddenly, changing everything it touches, and it takes a long time for everyone to put things together again afterward. Loss of a relationship, a job, or a way of life are also examples of catastrophic change.

Brain injury, too, is a traumatic event. It happens suddenly. It often has a catastrophic effect on the survivor and the survivor's family and friends. It takes a long time to heal. After brain injury, as after an earthquake, everything

Lynne says... Most people stay in shock for as long as they need to be protected from all the feelings they might be having about the brain injury. Many people take days or weeks before they start feeling the full impact of the trauma.

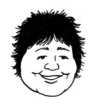

Lynne says...
A brain injury qualifies as a traumatic event whether or not it is called a traumatic brain injury or an acquired brain injury. What the injury is called is not important. What is important is the emotional impact.

changes. There are many losses, and nothing is ever exactly the same as it was again.

As a caregiver, you know that you, too, experienced trauma when your loved one did. Your life and your family's changed in an instant. After the brain injury happened, you might have first seen your loved one in an emergency ward of a hospital. Your loved one might have been disoriented or perhaps even unconscious. You and your family probably rearranged your lives to support your loved one. You lost the relationship you had with your loved one before the brain injury. Although you and your loved one have made many gains since the brain injury happened, you are probably also feeling some traumatic losses.

How does emotional recovery from trauma happen? Whether you're a caregiver or a survivor, recovering emotionally from the trauma of brain injury depends on these things:

- Some time has passed since the traumatic event so that healing can start.

- You feel ready to start working on psychological recovery.

- You feel safe enough to be aware of your feelings.

- You have help in dealing with your feelings.

You've already made a start at recovering emotionally by reading this book.

Core Issues in Emotional Recovery

Common core issues

Certain feelings come up for almost everyone who goes through a trauma like brain injury. Many healthcare providers call these core issues. Core issues are the topic of this section.

Everyone is unique, and everyone experiences trauma in their own way. However, in the time just after trauma happens, most people feel similar kinds of losses:

- The loss of cognitive adeptness, which is the ability to think and make decisions quickly and easily. Do you remember feeling foggy all the time?

- The loss of easy, smooth social interactions. With all the trauma that was in your life, you might have found yourself unable to chit-chat.

- The loss of family closeness or the capacity for intimacy. Everyone copes with trauma in their own way. Some families split apart, not wanting to bother each other with their own pain.

- The loss of independence. Whether this loss is yours or your loved one's, you feel it.

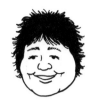

Lynne says... Dr. Janet Geringer Woititz, a specialist in addictions and emotional recovery, developed many important and instructive recovery materials. One of her many contributions was a list of common core issues* faced by trauma survivors. This list has been adapted to fit the experiences of survivors of brain injury and their caregivers.

* Janet Geringer Woititz, Adult Children of Alcoholics, published by Health Communications Inc., 1984, page 104. Used and adapted with permission.

After Brain Injury: Tools for Living
A Step-by-Step Guide for Caregivers and Survivors

What really matters is what happens in us — not to us.

ANONYMOUS

Loss is a core issue many people talk about, but it is not the only core issue in emotional recovery. Like many people, you probably also have some of these core issues:

- ❏ control
- ❏ intimacy
- ❏ courage
- ❏ willingness to grow
- ❏ emotional expression
- ❏ trust and safety
- ❏ denial
- ❏ self-reliance
- ❏ grieving
- ❏ healing the self

You might feel that these core issues are overwhelming. You might find it hard to imagine ever healing from them and feeling better. The good news is that over time, with patience and willingness, you *can* heal. The next main section of this book shows you a path to emotional recovery, taking one step at a time.

Before you move to that section, however, there is one other important issue to look at — trauma roles. Trauma roles are not usually called core issues, but do affect most people after they have experienced trauma, whether they are caregivers, survivors, or family and friends. Healing from trauma roles is an important part of emotional recovery.

Trauma roles

Understanding trauma roles

Following a trauma like brain injury, many people take on one or more of these trauma roles: Victim, Rescuer, and Persecutor.

What are trauma roles? Trauma roles are parts people take on automatically, without thinking about it, in hard times. These parts, or roles, help people get through the early time after trauma. Trauma roles give people something to do that helps them feel better in the emergency.

Trauma Roles*

Following a trauma like brain injury, many people take on one or more of these trauma roles.

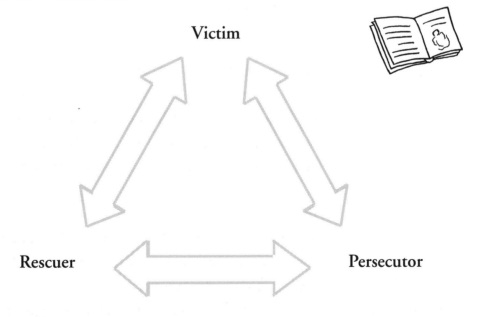

* In the early 1970s, drama therapist Stephen Karpman came up with the idea for the picture of the basic drama triangle you see here. It's now known as the Karpman Drama Triangle.

Adversity doesn't build character, it reveals it.

Anonymous

Victim-Rescuer-Persecutor roles often start in the early stages of recovery after brain injury. These roles develop as a result of circumstance and need. During the time when your loved one's life and level of disability are at stake, trauma roles comfort you and help you feel less anxious. These roles protect you from feeling too much anxiety.

You might find that you take on all three trauma roles at one time or another. You probably don't take on the same trauma role all the time with everyone. With your loved one, the survivor, you might take on the Rescuer role at one time and the Victim role at another. With your partner or spouse, you might take on the Rescuer role at one time and the Persecutor role at another. With a healthcare provider, you might take on the Victim role at one time and the Persecutor role at another. And so on.

Of course, caregivers like you aren't the only ones who take on these roles. You probably see your loved one and your family and friends taking on trauma roles, too. It's a normal reaction to too much upheaval and loss.

What do these trauma roles look like? The next section gives you some brief examples. Once you have read them, you can probably think of some examples from your own life.

Victim

In the Victim trauma role, you feel helpless and powerless to bring about any change. You are overwhelmed with pain and loss. You look to others for solutions to your problems. You probably blame yourself for all kinds of things.

Here's what someone in the Victim trauma role might sound like: "My loved one has a brain injury. We no longer have control over our lives. Things will probably never get better. I guess that's the way it is…unless a miracle happens. What can I do? I feel helpless."

"What can I do? I feel helpless."

Rescuer
In the Rescuer trauma role, you focus almost completely on the needs of others, as you perceive them. You feel driven to take care of those needs. You tell yourself that your help is needed and that it's a way you can feel useful. You do not allow yourself to feel or talk about your own feelings of pain, loss, or worry.

Here's what someone in the Rescuer trauma role might sound like: "Looking after myself is not important. Looking after my loved one is. My loved one is the one who counts. My loved one needs help. Whatever my loved one wants, I'll try to give it. It's good to be needed."

"My loved one is the one who counts."

Persecutor
In the Persecutor trauma role, you might turn into a kind of tyrant. You take over whatever you think needs to be done with your loved one and your family and friends to help them through this hard time. You plan and control. You tell people what to do. If they don't cooperate, you probably get angry with them. You drown out your own feelings by keeping busy and making sure that everyone else does, too.

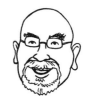

Mike says…
The first people in the hospital might say something like this: 'Take care of yourself. There is nothing you can do right now. Get some respite.' Inside you are feeling: 'There must be something I can do and need to do to make it better. He is my child!' That's how I began my Rescuer role.

Here's what someone in the Persecutor trauma role might sound like: "No one else knows what needs to be done. I have to look after everything myself. That's the only way I can cope with all this."

"No one else knows what needs to be done."

Letting go of trauma roles

Like denial and other core issues, trauma roles serve a purpose — they help you get through a hard time automatically, without much thinking. The trouble is, some people get stuck in their trauma roles. Long after the trauma first happened, they find it almost impossible to deal with things in any other way.

Getting stuck in a trauma role is like getting stuck in denial and other core issues. Like denial and other core issues, trauma roles can become stoppers to growth and healing. They become stoppers to the inner conversations between the Social Self and the Real Self. That's why letting go of trauma roles is an important part of emotional recovery.

The next main section of this book shows you the Five-Stage Emotional Recovery Model, which describes ways you can let go of trauma roles, denial, and other core issues and start recovering emotionally.

Before looking at the Five-Stage Recovery Model, now is a good time to pause and do the worksheet on the following pages:

- (3-1) Trauma Roles and Recovery Worksheet

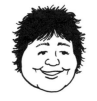

Lynne says... Even if you think you are not stuck in any trauma roles, ask a trusted friend for feedback.

Chapter 3: Recovering Emotionally
Core Issues in Emotional Recovery

Helping Your Survivor

Is Lack of Impulse Control an Emotional Problem?

One of the most frequent complaints of survivors of brain injury is their "short fuse," their inability to control their impulses. These survivors often act before they think, then later feel regret about their actions. They also feel confused about what to do next. They can't figure out how to act more appropriately.

As a caregiver, you might have seen this kind of behavior in your loved one. When you start helping your loved one with emotional recovery, it might help to know that her/his lack of impulse control is a cognitive disability. This inability for survivors to practice proper anger management is often mistaken for an emotional problem.

If your loved one's lack of impulse control is a problem for you, look in Chapter 2 and in the Resources section at the end of this book for the SST (Stop-Still-Think) Instructional Aid and use it to help you.

SST is based on the idea that it's not the emotions that need attention, but the lack of impulse control. The survivor's outbursts may not be psychologically meaningful at all. They may be impulses, which are, for the moment, untrained. The SST aid helps interrupt the impulsive cycle, empowering the survivor to control his/her "short fuse" and improve social skills and interpersonal relations.

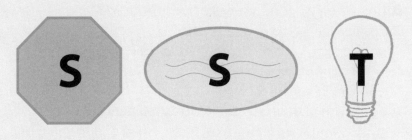

After Brain Injury: Tools for Living
A Step-by-Step Guide for Caregivers and Survivors

W 3-1

Trauma Roles and Recovery Worksheet

Read the descriptions of the "I am…when I" trauma roles below and decide which role you take on most often. Put a checkmark beside each statement that is true for you. Then look at the "I can stop" list that follows. This list will give you examples of

I am in the victim role when I: *(Check any that are true for you.)*
- ❏ let other people do things for me and make plans for me
- ❏ believe that there is nothing I can do to change my own life
- ❏ don't believe I can get any of my needs met
- ❏ believe I am inferior to others and should step aside for them
- ❏ let other people make important decisions for me
- ❏ don't take responsibility for my own life
- ❏ avoid conflict and think I wouldn't get what I want anyway
- ❏ remain quiet about issues or feelings that are important to me
- ❏ expect others to hurt or disappoint me

I am rescuing when I: *(Check any that are true for you.)*
- ❏ do something I really don't want to do
- ❏ say "yes" when I mean "no"
- ❏ do something for someone even though that person is capable of doing it and should be doing it himself/herself
- ❏ meet people's needs without being asked and before I've agreed to do so
- ❏ do more than my fair share of work after my help is requested
- ❏ consistently give more than I receive in a particular situation
- ❏ fix other people's feelings
- ❏ do other people's thinking for them

I am persecuting when I: *(Check any that are true for you.)*
- ❏ tell other people what to do or give orders
- ❏ put other people down, make fun of them, or call people names
- ❏ invalidate other people's experiences
- ❏ manipulate others to get what I want
- ❏ control the behavior of others by threats or intimidation
- ❏ withhold my love and support from others as a way of punishing or intimidating them
- ❏ believe my own feelings and ideas are more important than anyone else's
- ❏ actively blame others for my own situation

what it would look like if you stopped taking on that particular role. Check off one thing on each list that you will start working on now.

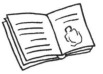

I can stop being a victim by: *(Check one that you will start working on now.)*
- educating myself on the difference between the victim role and the experience of victimization
- validating my own experiences, yet expanding my choices of how to respond to situations
- learning life skills such as assertiveness, communication and stress reduction
- seeking out people who will encourage a positive image of myself
- changing the circumstances that result in my feeling a victim
- breaking down my isolation

I can stop rescuing by: *(Check one that you will start working on now.)*
- limiting myself to doing no more than 50 per cent of the work in any relationship
- believing that others are not helpless
- giving others the information and support that can help them in changing their own lives
- being honest about my own feelings, needs and wants
- learning to separate my "need to be needed" from my genuine caring and compassion
- learning to set limits with others and to improve my feelings about myself
- identifying my own feelings, needs and wants

I can stop persecuting by: *(Check one that you will start working on now.)*
- learning to identify my feelings of anger
- finding suitable outlets for my feelings that are not hurtful to others
- using communication and assertion skills as an alternate way of communicating my thoughts and feelings
- learning to identify my feelings, needs, and wants
- working to feel better about myself
- remembering that it is my behavior that is the problem, not me or my feelings or needs

[The material on these two pages was written by a creative soul whose name could not be traced. Thanks!]

After Brain Injury: Tools for Living
A Step-by-Step Guide for Caregivers and Survivors

The Five-Stage Emotional Recovery Model

This section presents the Five-Stage Emotional Recovery Model, a program worked out to help people recover emotionally from trauma — people like you and your loved one. First, you will look briefly at what makes up the five stages that most people experience while recovering emotionally from trauma. Second, you will have a chance to explore these stages in more detail and understand where you are in your own emotional recovery.

Look closely at the Five-Stage Emotional Recovery Model pictured. You will probably see parts that look familiar.

Stages of Emotional Recovery

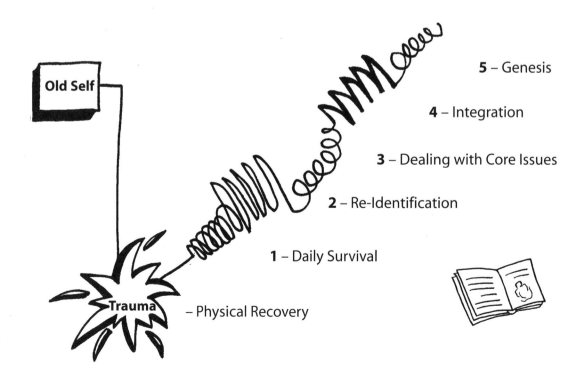

Chapter 3: Recovering Emotionally
The Five-Stage Emotional Recovery Model

First, look at the part labeled Old Self. This part refers to the Psychological Self as it was before the trauma happened. A line connecting the Old Self to the Trauma shows the loss or unbalancing of Self that often happens with trauma.

Next, look at Physical Recovery. You might wonder why it is there. This part was added because, like most caregivers, you focused first on the survivor's physical recovery after brain injury.

You probably remember many things about the time it took for your loved one to start to recover and heal physically. At first, there were probably many exciting signs of physical recovery. Gradually, however, physical recovery probably slowed down. Healing and growth was still happening, and would continue to happen for a long time, but it happened just a bit at a time. You probably recognize this as the stage when you and your loved one started focusing on other things, such as recovering emotionally from the trauma.

Next, look at the five spirals. Each is a stage in emotional recovery. Why spirals? Recovering emotionally isn't often as simple as moving up in a straight line and never going back down to a previous stage. Instead, emotional recovery sometimes involves going back to an earlier stage where it feels safer. When the Psychological Self is recovering, you need to grow in safe steps. Each time you don't feel safe, your Psychological Self will automatically return you to the Daily Survival level of recovery.

Lynne says... The emotional recovery model we use in this chapter is not a new one. It was developed in the 1950s and was first used with adults who were recovering from substance abuse. Since then, the model has been used in many types of trauma recovery programs. In the 1980s, we began using this model in our recovery program for survivors of trauma like you and your loved one.

Finally, look at the five stages. Each stage is different and involves particular issues, feelings, and thoughts, as well as unique challenges and changes. Here's a brief summary of each stage:

Stage 1 – Daily Survival

You just make it through every day. You feel both worry and hope. You constantly ask yourself the question: Who am I, now?

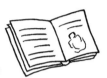

Stage 2 – Re-Identification

You find a name for the problem or challenge you are facing. This naming needs to feel right or true for you. You might have to try out many names before one feels true.

Stage 3 – Dealing with Core Issues

You are able to make change happen. This kind of action is sometimes called the operant level of change. This is the level of change that other people can see.

Stage 4 – Integration

Negatives become positives. Liabilities become assets. You start to appreciate the struggle of recovery and the learning that comes with it.

Stage 5 – Genesis

You start to contribute to the world in specific ways. You go beyond the concerns of your self.

Exploring the Five-Stage Emotional Recovery Model in more detail

After seeing the short descriptions of the five stages in the emotional recovery model, you probably already have feelings, thoughts, and ideas about each one, based on your own experience. This section is your chance to explore the five stages — and your responses to them — in more detail.

Stage 1 – Daily Survival

In the first stage of emotional recovery, the most important thing you do is survive the pressures of the day. Just making it through the day is the one and only goal you can achieve at this first level of healing.

Like most caregivers, you probably felt shock at the Daily Survival stage. You might feel numb now. You might feel as if you are always waiting and worrying. You probably hope that someone will help you find solutions to all the problems. You might think that if only someone could find a solution, you wouldn't worry so much.

At this stage, the automatic protection mechanism of denial shows up and does its work. As you will remember from Chapter 2, denial helps you cope when there is too much loss and upheaval in your life and your Real Self does not feel safe. Early on, you go into shock so that you won't be overwhelmed. You do only what you need to do to survive — whatever that is. Denial is not conscious. That means:

- You don't need to be aware of denial for it to appear.

- You don't decide to do it or have it.

There are no hopeless situations — only people who are hopeless about them.

DINAH SHORE

The automatic protection mechanism of denial helps you set aside most of your feelings and get through a hard time. In the Daily Survival stage, this denial usually has some extra features. You might find yourself doing a certain behavior over and over just to make it through the day — or the moment. You might feel as though you're stuck. You might wait for others to tell you what to do next, even when they seem unable to do so.

How can you tell whether you're in the Daily Survival stage of denial? Ask yourself: "How am I, right now?" Then look at this list and check off what applies to you:

❑ I set aside most of my feelings just to get through the day.

❑ I have no words for my feelings.

❑ I find myself doing a certain behavior over and over just to make it through the day — or the moment.

❑ I feel as though I'm stuck.

❑ I'm waiting and hoping for someone to tell me what to do next.

If most of the things in this list feel true for you, you are not yet ready to move to the second stage of recovery. You probably are just where you need to be to feel safe. Remember that safety comes first. Safety is absolutely necessary for growth to happen. You must feel safe inside and outside before you can start to let go of shock and denial.

Chapter 3: Recovering Emotionally
The Five-Stage Emotional Recovery Model

Even after you have moved on to the other stages of emotional recovery, you might find that you return to the Daily Survival stage once in a while. This is normal. This is a safe place to be until you re-identify, once again, your need to grow.

That is why we have put spirals in the picture of the Five-Stage Emotional Recovery Model. The spirals show that recovery is not a straight line. You will likely need to return to the Daily Survival stage each and every time you feel too much anxiety. There you can rest, gather courage, and build up your willingness to start growing again. Then once again you can move up to Re-Identification and onward.

Sometimes shock and denial fade gradually, and sometimes they stop all at once. It's as though you suddenly wake up. Usually that's when two things have started happening. Until these two things start happening, you will wait, worry, and hope that someone else can come up with ideas that will solve your problems. You will get frustrated because there are no magic solutions. You will return again and again to numbness and worry. What are these important two things?

1. You realize that your recovery is up to you. You know that you can ask others for help, but only you can find solutions.

2. You start to have an attitude of willingness. As you saw in Chapter 2, willingness is being ready to take a risk and learn something new. Willingness allows you to be curious, open, and exploring even when you feel scared or frustrated.

If I had my life to live over I would have gone to bed when I was sick instead of pretending the earth would go into a holding pattern if I weren't there for the day.

Erma Bombeck

Once you have realized that your recovery is up to you and have started to have an attitude of willingness, you're probably already in the second stage of emotional recovery, which is called Re-Identification.

Helping Your Survivor

Everyone Is Different

Your loved one, too, may be in Daily Survival, the first stage of emotional recovery. Or your loved one may still be almost completely focused on physical recovery. Whatever stage your loved one is in, that's where he/she needs to be. Don't expect both of you to be at the same stage of emotional recovery. That would be unusual, since emotional recovery is a healing process that is different for each person.

Stage 2 – Re-Identification

After the shock and denial of the first stage of emotional recovery start to fade, you start to be able to name your feelings. At this second stage of emotional recovery, most people name their feelings as loss.

In this second stage, whatever you were thinking or feeling about loss in the Daily Survival stage changes. You give your experience a new name, one that re-identifies the experience in some way. You experience a change in how you understand what is going on inside yourself. In turn, this change inside you affects how you see those around you and what you expect of them.

How do you know you're in this stage? You feel a shift. You move from not being able to name your loss, or even feel

Chapter 3: Recovering Emotionally
The Five-Stage Emotional Recovery Model

it, to giving your experience a name. Once you begin searching for your own names for your experience, you have entered this stage. If a new name helps you understand yourself and if it feels true, then you're in the Re-Identification stage. Here's an example:

- You focus mostly on this thought: "My loved one has had a brain injury." You worry, and hope that the brain injury gets better. You're in the Daily Survival stage.

- Some time later, you have this thought: "Actually, my whole family has experienced the trauma of this brain injury and been affected by it." Now you're in the Re-Identification stage.

In the Re-Identification stage, you start asking yourself, "What's going on inside of me now?" And, because you're ready and because you're having inner conversations again, some part of you starts answering the question. You will know the exact moment when you have arrived in the Re-Identification stage because you can name exactly how you feel in one moment and the name feels just right. It is the feeling of "just right" that helps you recognize the Re-Identification stage.

How do Daily Survival and Re-Identification work in your own life? The following two sections take you through some of the experiences many caregivers have in the Daily Survival stage. Of course, your experience is different from anyone else's, but it might help you to see that others have experiences similar to yours in these first two stages of emotional recovery.

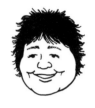

Lynne says ...
Re-Identification means finding new names for old challenges and problems. The emotional recovery process doesn't just work on what happened to you during the trauma. It works on problems and challenges you had before the trauma and helps you heal.

The Recovery Model described in this section is based on the works of Stephanie Brown, Herbert Gravitz and Julie Bowden. We use it here with their permission.

Take time to relax, especially when you don't have time for it.

Sydney J. Harris

Looking at Daily Survival in your own life

In the time after the brain injury happened, healthcare providers focused on your loved one's physical recovery in two ways:

- They worked to bring back as many of the survivor's physical abilities and skills as possible.

- They worked to reduce any disabilities connected with the brain injury.

These healthcare providers saw you at the hospital. They probably tried to comfort you. They understood that you were changing your routines to match the needs of your loved one. If they saw that you looked tired, they probably gave you well-meaning advice, such as: "Go home and try to get some sleep. We'll call you if anything changes. You need the rest."

In the time after the trauma, it might help for others to tell you to take care of yourself like this. You can probably not hear, identify, or name your self-care needs such as sleeping, eating, and simply resting. Like many caregivers, you might get used to not paying attention to your own needs. You get swept up in all the details of supporting your loved one.

New routines are imposed on you and your family by the trauma. You don't choose these routines, and they don't seem part of you. Your normal daily routines disappear and are replaced with emergency routines and schedules. You eat because there is a moment to eat, not because you feel hungry. You sleep because someone tells you to, not because you feel tired.

Chapter 3: Recovering Emotionally
The Five-Stage Emotional Recovery Model

Months or years later, you might find yourself overextended, doing more than you have time or energy to do. The "emergency" routines have become normal routines, whether your loved one is at home, in the hospital, or at the rehab center. You might find yourself sleeping poorly and not eating properly. You might have sudden emotional outbreaks, such as bursting into tears. You don't yet realize the full effect on yourself and your family of supporting your loved one.

It is also quite possible that your lack of appetite and poor sleep habits are at least partly the result of depression. If your doctor suggests that you are showing the classic signs of depression, you may not even react. You may not feel much of anything. You can't identify yourself as depressed. You just want to get through the day and do what you have to do. This is what Daily Survival is like.

The butterfly counts not months but moments, and has time enough.

RABINDRANATH TAGORE

Remember that this is your book. You might want to pause here and write a bit about what Daily Survival is like for you.

I know I am in Daily Survival when . . .

_____

_____

_____

_____

After Brain Injury: Tools for Living
A Step-by-Step Guide for Caregivers and Survivors

The truth will set you free ... but first, it will make you miserable.

ANONYMOUS

Looking at Re-Identification in your own life

With time, and when you're ready, you realize that your recovery is up to you. You start having an attitude of willingness. That's when you start to shift from Daily Survival to Re-Identification.

Maybe the shift happens this way.... Imagine you're on your way home from the doctor's office one day. You notice two children playing in the park. One child grabs the other's toy and runs away. You suddenly start crying and you have this thought: "I feel sad. I want my loved one back the way they were." You continue crying.

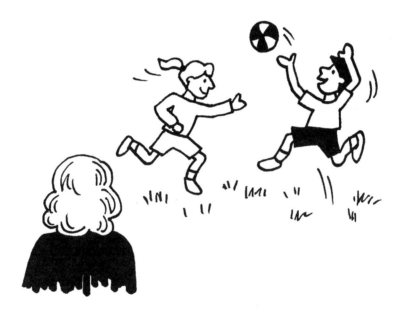

You have just re-identified depression as loss, longing, or sorrow. This is the Re-Identification stage. For the first time in a long time, the language you are using fits with how you feel. For maybe just those few moments, you feel whole again. You may not be happy, but you are whole. Your Social self and your Real Self are communicating well. What you are thinking and feeling outside matches what you are thinking and feeling inside.

Chapter 3: Recovering Emotionally
The Five-Stage Emotional Recovery Model

In the Re-Identification stage, you will probably have many experiences like this. Gradually you will realize that you are changing. You are no longer numb, frozen — even though much still needs to heal. You no longer try to make other people's labels fit your experience. You are becoming much more open to recognizing your situation as it really is. You are having inner conversations again. You are probably ready to start dealing with your core issues.

Stage 3 – Dealing with Core Issues

At the Re-Identification stage, you realize that the term "loss" describes your experience. If you continue listening carefully to yourself with respect, you enter the next stage of emotional recovery and start dealing with loss and your other core issues.

In order to hear exactly what you must do at this stage, you need to listen carefully and often to your Real Self. This is when all the work you've done to have inner conversations really pays off.

One part of that work was making yourself aware of your own negative, judgmental self-talk, then practicing positive self-talk. Now you can listen to your Psychological Self without judgment, and that brings about another shift. What is this shift? As you get better at listening to yourself, you also start listening with openness and acceptance rather than with judgment and impatience. You need this important ability in order to deal with your core issues.

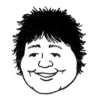

Lynne says … Much of the healing of your loss or any of the common core issues in recovery has a lot to do with not getting in your own way. You need to listen to yourself as if you expect to hear something important.

> Most people deal with core issues like these:
>
> loss
>
> control
>
> intimacy
>
> courage
>
> willingness to grow
>
> emotional expression
>
> trust
>
> denial
>
> safety
>
> self-reliance
>
> grieving
>
> healing the self

Go back, for a moment, to the earlier section where you imagined re-identifying your loss while watching two children play. One child takes something from the other child. You put yourself in that picture as the person naming your own loss, perhaps for the first time. What you are thinking and feeling outside matches what you are thinking and feeling inside. In that moment, the name you use to describe your loss feels exactly right and true for you. At this point you have two choices:

- You can ignore your newly recognized truth or choose not to hold on to it. You can push it back by using negative, judgmental self-talk, such as "Look at silly me, crying outside in front of the world."

OR

- You can hold on to your newly recognized truth carefully, with respect.

What are the consequences of these choices?

- If you judge yourself and your experience negatively, your Real Self hides and stops communicating with you. You move away from knowing and feeling more. Your loss once again becomes buried deep inside you. This may be what you need to do to feel safe.

- If you respect your experience and hold it carefully in front of you, you validate it. You feel it as true for you. You also allow yourself to feel the full emotional impact of your experience. You accept that this will hurt for a while.

Chapter 3: Recovering Emotionally
The Five-Stage Emotional Recovery Model

If you can hold your experience and respect it, you put yourself in the psychological position of being open and willing to listen to yourself. From that position, you can learn even more about yourself and what you need. If you listen respectfully and often enough, one day the thing you need to do for your emotional recovery will become clear to you. At that time, you might find yourself saying something like this:

A closed mind is a good thing to lose.

ANONYMOUS

"I need to do _____[this]_____ about my loss."

The "this" could be many things. Here are a few examples:

"I need to . . ."

- "I need to cry and accept my crying as an expression of my loss."

- "I need to allow myself to grieve."

- "I need to talk to my very best friend about this."

- "I need to allow the word 'loss' to exist inside me."

- "I need to find a safe person with whom I can explore my loss."

It's as though your Real Self is giving you instructions about what you need to do to heal and grow and stay safe. If you follow these inner instructions, you will be on the path to healing your core issues, whatever they may be, and moving into the fourth stage of emotional recovery — Integration.

The Chinese word for "crisis" contains two characters. One of them means "opportunity."

Anonymous

Stage 4 – Integration

Moving through the first three stages of emotional recovery from trauma — from numb worry (Daily Survival) to naming (Re-Identification) to dealing with the loss (Dealing with Core Issues) — involves more than enough pain for anyone. The good news is that once you pass through these three stages, you will find that your pain is already lessening.

If you let these first three stages take place in the way and time that is just right for you, positive changes will start to happen. The biggest change you will notice is that what you used to feel was a liability, a problem, starts to become an asset, something positive. When this happens, you have reached the Integration stage of emotional recovery.

Here's how it often happens. During the third stage of emotional recovery, you've been dealing with loss and other core issues. One day, after one more honest grieving experience about loss, you find yourself saying something like this to yourself (or to someone else): "If I had never acknowledged this loss and experienced all the grief that came with it, I would never have grown into the _____ person that I am becoming." What you put in the blank space will be unique to you.

Here are some other examples of statements you might make in the Integration stage:

- "Feeling my grief made me more tolerant of others and my own imperfections."

- "Facing my own losses allowed me to have fun again."

- "Sharing my sadness with others brought me closer to everyone in my family. I stopped keeping secrets."

- "Accepting my loss has allowed me to see my loved one differently too."

What used to feel like trauma, loss and difficulty now feels like a positive gain or strength. Maybe you're already moving into the fifth stage of recovery — Genesis.

Stage 5 – Genesis

You worry and hope your way through the Daily Survival stage. At the Re-Identification stage, you start to feel that you are getting a handle on what seemed unknowable to you before. In the Dealing with Core Issues stage, you face whatever you need to face in order to recover from trauma. Then, in the Integration stage, you recognize that strengths and assets can come out of trauma.

Like most people, you probably stay in the Integration stage for a while. You need time to experience what this new awareness of strengths and assets feels like. You need time to become used to looking at yourself as someone who has strengths and assets. Only then can you start to see that the larger world needs those strengths and assets. You start to feel ready to make a new beginning. This readiness for a new beginning is known as Genesis, the fifth and final stage in the Emotional Recovery Model.

By this time, you have learned valuable lessons. You started by realizing that your recovery is up to you. You decided to

Mike says . . .
Facing my own losses has allowed me to be more honest about the way I feel. While I may never say all these feelings aloud, I notice the change inside me. I also now realize it's okay to bounce back and forth between these stages. I'm getting comfortable with that.

People say that walking on water is a miracle, but to me walking peacefully on earth is the real miracle.

Benjamin Disraeli

develop an attitude of willingness so that change could happen. You worked through the stages of emotional recovery. Sometimes you needed to go back to earlier stages for a while. You learned to go at your own pace.

You also learned from your loss and pain. Maybe you learned how to accept and value others — even in challenging situations. Maybe you learned ways to stay patient and understanding. You have allowed change to prepare you to contribute to the world in new and positive ways.

The lessons you have learned are valuable not only for you, but for others. You probably now have the extra energy and skills to help the world outside you. You have things to share with others about your experience. You know that your sharing will also help your own ongoing healing. You know how to take care of yourself. You're ready to support your

Be Kind To Yourself

Remember that emotional recovery takes place slowly over time. You recover bit by bit, core issue by core issue, stage by stage. Keep in mind that you may not move through the various stages of emotional recovery as quickly as you want. Be kind to yourself. Know that you may find yourself going back to previous stages whenever you feel overwhelmed and upset or need to rest.

loved one, your family, your community, and society in a truly healthy way.

The attitude within is more important than the circumstances without.

ANONYMOUS

Now is a good time to pause and do the worksheet on the following page:

- (3-2) Identifying My Issues in Emotional Recovery

This worksheet will help you identify some of your core issues and think about where you are in the five stages of emotional recovery.

After you have done this worksheet, you will be ready for the last two chapters in the book. In these chapters, you will notice a change from the focus on self and emotional recovery to a focus on recovery in thinking and behavior. Another change you will notice: The next two chapters apply more to your loved one than to you, the caregiver, but give you practical tools that you can both use to start thinking in new ways and changing behavior.

After Brain Injury: Tools for Living
A Step-by-Step Guide for Caregivers and Survivors

W 3-2

Identifying My Issues in Emotional Recovery

Below is a list of common core issues that people like you, who have experienced trauma, have identified. Look at the issues in the list below. Pick one issue that feels most relevant to you, today in this moment. Try not to think too much about which one you choose. There is no right or wrong answer.

Control	Healing denial through safety
Intimacy	Dealing with changed cognition
Courage and willingness to grow	Self-reliance
Emotional expression	Loss and grieving
Learning to trust again	Healing the self

1. Write the issue you have identified here: _____

2. Using the Five-Stage Emotional Recovery Model, identify your present stage of recovery for this issue:

   ❏ I am stuck, worried, and waiting. (Daily Survival stage)
   ❏ I have just re-identified this issue by naming it. While it may make me anxious, it feels exactly like the experience I am having. (Re-Identification stage)
   ❏ I am practicing a new response or behavior each time this issue happens. (Core Issues stage)
   ❏ While this issue was difficult to process, I am now a better...[problem-solver, person, negotiator]...because of facing it. (Integration stage)
   ❏ After working on recovery on this issue, I now know I have something to offer. I can contribute by...[volunteering, getting politically active, advocating]. (Genesis stage)

3. How will you keep track of your recovery work on this issue?

   ❏ I will journal daily and review my writing weekly.
   ❏ I will tell a friend about my journey in recovery.
   ❏ I will share my work with myself, tolerating change and the anxiety and hope it brings.
   ❏ I will review and redo this exercise weekly.

4. Your own ideas:
   ❏ _____
   ❏ _____

5. Decide on one action to do this week and write it here:
   _____
   _____

4 Thinking in New Ways

Learning goals for this chapter

This chapter looks at how you can help your loved one start thinking in new ways as part of his/her recovery from a brain injury. First, this chapter helps you understand how certain parts of the brain work and how they affect thinking. Second, this chapter looks at strategies and tools for helping your loved one learn six important thinking skills. These strategies will help your loved one deal with her/his cognitive disabilities and help you both feel less overwhelmed by them.

In this chapter, you will have a chance to:

- understand common cognitive disabilities better
- learn about the brain, especially the frontal lobe of the brain and its role in thinking
- use practical tools for guiding the thinking process in a person with brain injury

Introduction

Right now I'm having amnesia and déjà vu *at the same time. I think I've forgotten this before.*

ANONYMOUS

The first three chapters of this book have been based on the fact that when the brain injury happened, two things took place:

- First, your loved one experienced physical trauma. You did what you could to support your loved one is her/his physical recovery.

- Second, both you and your loved one experienced psychological trauma. You both needed to go through many of the same steps for psychological recovery. If you have been working through this book, by now you both probably understand the Psychological Self better, have started to have inner conversations again, and are moving through the stages of emotional recovery.

All this has prepared you for the last two steps in psychological recovery — thinking in new ways and changing behavior. These are the topics of this chapter and Chapter 5.

You will notice that these last two chapters of the book shift gears a bit. They focus more on experiences that are common for survivors of brain injury. However, in these chapters you will increase your understanding of thinking and behavior and look at tools that help start new ways of thinking and behaving. You can use this knowledge to help your loved one. In the process, you might also apply this knowledge to your own thinking and behavior.

You will find a number of worksheets in this chapter. They all show a logical, step-by-step process for learning certain cognitive skills. You will find that you need more than one worksheet for each cognitive skill. Once you have filled in the worksheets in this chapter, go to the Resources section at the end of this book and photocopy extra worksheets. Place the worksheets in file folders that you have labeled (for example, Project-Planning, Decision-Making) and store the files where you can see and find them easily.

What does thinking include?

Many healthcare providers use the word "thinking" when they talk about the brain and the mind. You've probably heard this word often since your loved one survived brain injury.

You might also have heard healthcare providers use the word "cognition." Cognition is how the brain and the mind work together to do many important tasks, called cognitive functions. Cognitive functions include tasks like these:

- receiving and organizing information from the senses

- being aware of self

- predicting results of actions

- organizing thoughts

- managing time and energy

- planning and organizing activities

> There are five senses: seeing, touching, hearing, tasting, smelling.
>
> All these senses provide information for thinking.

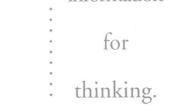

If you don't do it, you'll never know what would have happened if you had done it.

ASHLEIGH BRILLIANT

- setting goals

- solving problems

- making decisions

- concentrating on a certain task

- doing or thinking more than one thing at a time (multi-tasking)

- remembering

Why focus on thinking?

Everything humans do is guided, controlled, created or allowed by the brain. An injury to the brain therefore most often affects thinking. In turn, thinking affects many other things, such as sense of self or identity, physical mobility, perception and sensation, and personality.

Because it affects so much, many survivors and caregivers identify thinking as a very important issue in recovery. Survivors say that they have difficulties especially with these three cognitive functions: memory, concentration, and being aware of themselves.

Changed self-awareness can be one of the most important effects of brain injury. It prevents survivors from being able to notice or fully describe their disability.

You probably notice that your loved one has cognitive difficulties in addition to the ones just listed. Many caregivers say that the survivor they care for and about has difficulties in planning, setting goals and carrying them out, judging, problem-solving, decision-making, maintaining attention and focus, multi-track thinking and multi-tasking, and getting and staying organized.

An injury to the brain might affect the person for a short time or for a lifetime. After brain injury, the person might need to learn to think all over again or think in new ways. That's the focus of this chapter.

The Brain and How It Affects Thinking

Main parts of the brain

The main parts of the brain are these: four lobes (frontal, temporal, occipital, and parietal) and cerebellum. Each part of the brain carries out specific jobs, or functions, as the chart on the next page shows.

The frontal lobe as a conductor

While all the parts of the brain are needed, this section focuses on the frontal lobe, which is particularly important as the executive control center of the brain.

Imagine the conductor of a symphony orchestra. The conductor decides on the music the orchestra will play, arranges the music as needed to suit the orchestra's abilities and needs, and leads the orchestra in practicing and performing the music.

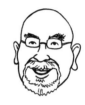

Mike says . . . Book-mark this section. It's not you, and not your loved one who makes mistakes. It's the frontal lobe trying as hard as it can. This analogy of the frontal lobe as a conductor is easy for me to follow and explains why my loved one can't focus on conversations or on more than one activity at a time.

The Brain's Jobs

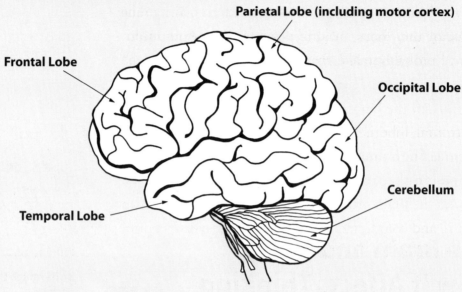

Part	Job
frontal lobe	Also called the executive control center, it's the conductor of the brain. Controls personality, curiosity, planning, problem-solving, higher-order thinking, and emotional restraint.
temporal lobe	Interprets sound and speech; deals with some aspects of long-term memory.
occipital lobe	Handles what the eyes see.
parietal lobe	Deals with orientation, calculation, and makes certain types of recognition possible, such as face recognition.
cerebellum	Monitors impulses from nerve endings in the muscles. Coordinates the smoothness of every movement in the body. Important in the learning, performance and timing of complex motor tasks, including speaking.

This chart was adapted from How the Special Needs Brain Learns, *by David A. Sousa. Thousand Oaks, CA: Corwin Press, 2001, page 8.*

Chapter 4: Thinking in New Ways
The Brain and How It Affects Thinking

After the orchestra performs a concert, the conductor gives the players feedback on their overall performance and gives individual players specific feedback about their playing. The conductor then starts making plans for the next concert, and will probably make changes to the music and to the players.

The frontal lobe is like the conductor of a symphony orchestra. The frontal lobe organizes and coordinates all the information that the brain collects, uses, and produces. Injury to the brain often affects the frontal lobe's ability to organize and coordinate, as well as other executive control functions like planning and problem-solving.

The frontal lobe also houses the self-will area, which some people call the personality. This area includes curiosity and

The Frontal Lobe as a Conductor

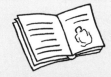

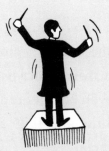

The frontal lobe is like the conductor of a symphony orchestra. The conductor decides, arranges, and leads. After a performance, the conductor gives feedback, makes changes, and plans the next performance.

After an injury to the brain, the frontal lobe's ability to organize and coordinate is affected. When the frontal lobe can no longer work well from inside, tools and strategies from outside the brain can help.

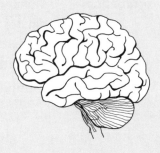

If you tell the truth you don't have to remember anything.

ANONYMOUS

the ability to express and control emotions. As a result, injury to the frontal lobe of the brain might not only affect thinking skills, but also change personality and behavior. Like all cognitive functions affected by brain injury, these changes might last a short time or a lifetime.

When the frontal lobe is injured and can no longer work well from the inside, tools and strategies from outside can help. Many of the tools and strategies described in the next section act as helpers to the frontal lobe.

Strategies and Tools for Learning Six Thinking Skills

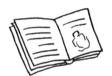

This section focuses on six important thinking skills that most survivors of brain injury find difficult to do: (1) setting goals, (2) making decisions, (3) doing a task analysis, (4) solving problems, (5) planning projects, and (6) managing time and energy.

Learning or relearning each skill involves using certain strategies and tools, such as worksheets and memory aids. These strategies and tools will not make your loved one's difficulties go away, but will make you both more aware of what's involved in these important thinking skills and give your loved one practice in doing them.

While learning these strategies and tools, keep these important ideas in mind:

- Involve as many senses in learning as you can. Write out your thoughts. Draw pictures of how you think.

Chapter 4: Thinking in New Ways
Strategies and Tools for Learning Six Thinking Skills

- Break down your tasks into small, easy-to-do steps. Each step you do successfully will increase your confidence.

- Work on content first; worry about speed later.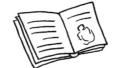

- Learn one new skill at a time.

- If you are deciding something important to you, look for a validator before you act. A validator is someone who will listen and give you feedback about your plan.

Someone who thinks logically is a nice contrast to the real world.

ANONYMOUS

(1) Setting goals

Goal-setting is one of those frontal lobe thinking skills that involves planning ahead and imagining results. Like most people, you probably find that setting goals is an important activity in your life. Setting goals is something you might do before you begin to make changes in your life. Having goals also helps after you have made changes. By looking back at the goals you set, you can tell whether you have changed and by how much.

Setting a goal means planning a pathway that is yours and right for you. You do not probably spend much time setting goals that aren't important for you. The same is true for your loved one.

When you plan a goal, you probably go through a process something like this: You set a hazy, vague goal. You start clarifying your goal. You finalize the goal by announcing it or writing it down.

Be not afraid of growing slowly, be afraid only of standing still.

CHINESE PROVERB

Of course the process of setting goals involves much more than these three simple steps. For example, you might think aloud or talk with someone else or write lists. That way, you get to try out some ideas by talking or thinking about them, then use these ideas in your planning.

Until now, you might have just gone through this goal-setting process automatically, without thinking about it much. The strategy for helping a person with a brain injury set goals is for you to look first at just how you go about setting goals.

Now is a good time to pause and do this worksheet:

- (4-1) Clear Goal-Setting Worksheet

It will help you understand how you set goals. After you have done this worksheet, you will be better prepared to teach this valuable cognitive skill to your loved one.

The Six Elements of a Good Goal

A good goal must be

1. important to you
2. able to be put into words
3. realistic for *you* to do
4. clear and focused (no alternatives)
5. countable
6. worth celebrating when it's achieved

W 4–1

Chapter 4: Thinking in New Ways
Strategies and Tools for Learning Six Thinking Skills

Clear Goal-Setting Worksheet

1. A Hazy Goal is a vague sense of something that you want — something you hope for. State your Hazy Goal:
   _____

2. Ask yourself whether your Hazy Goal is:

   ❑ personally important (Do I want to attain this goal?)
   ❑ achievable (Is this goal possible?)
   ❑ realistic (Can I do it?)
   ❑ measurable or countable (It must be, in order to work.)

   Then ask yourself: Does my Hazy Goal have alternatives, such as "Either I do this or I do that"? If so, choose one.

3. Does your Hazy Goal give you ways of measuring or counting your progress? How will you measure or count your progress?
   _____
   _____

4. What materials do you need for measuring your progress?
   _____
   _____

5. Describe the reward or celebration you plan when you succeed in reaching your goal.
   _____
   _____

6. Do you plan to achieve this goal by a certain time?
   No _____
   Yes, I plan to achieve this goal by _____ (insert the date here)

(2) Making decisions effectively

I'd love to make up my mind, but I can't remember where I left it.

ANONYMOUS

Have you ever had more than one goal, more than one possible choice you could make? Remember what it was like to weigh the pros and cons, trying to figure out what to do? Effective decision-making means making an informed decision: looking at wants, needs, and possible consequences — positive as well as negative — before taking action. For example, if you were looking at going back to school, you might think about each of these possible decisions: going to school full-time, going to school part-time, or auditing one course and seeing how you do.

Many people would find it very hard to make a decision from these three possibilities. A person with a brain injury would find it especially hard. These decisions often happen quickly, in response to an impulse or whim, based on just a bit of information. Sometimes the person with a brain injury does use a decision-making process, but it is too simple to suit the situation. That person's process works something like this: "I want...something. I see a way that I think I can get it. I do the thing that I feel like doing."

The strategy for helping a person with a brain injury make effective decisions is to make the process clear. Now is a good time to pause and do this worksheet:

- (4-2) Effective Decision-Making Worksheet

It will help you understand how you go about making informed decisions. After you have done this worksheet, you will be better prepared to teach this valuable cognitive skill to your loved one.

Chapter 4: Thinking in New Ways
Strategies and Tools for Learning Six Thinking Skills

Effective Decision-Making Worksheet

1. Think about the decision you are making. Write it down here:
   _____

2. List the other decisions you could make:

   A. I could _____

   OR
   B. I could _____

   OR
   C. I could _____

3. For each of the other decisions you could make, list the possible consequences, both negative and positive:

A.	B.	C.
positive consequences	positive consequences	positive consequences
_____	_____	_____
_____	_____	_____
negative consequences	negative consequences	negative consequences
_____	_____	_____
_____	_____	_____

4. Think carefully about the positive and negative consequences, then choose the best decision for you. Write down your best decision here:
   _____
   _____
   _____
   _____

(3) Doing a task analysis

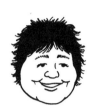

**Lynne says...
It's important to take the time to truly understand task analysis because many thinking aids are based on it. Once you truly get the process, you can design any tool you need. Because we cannot list and define all the skills your loved one will need to re-learn, you will need to understand how to build your own task analysis.**

When you are not sure what you need to learn or think about, task analysis can help in two ways: (1) before making a decision and (2) after making a decision, to plan a next step.

Task analysis involves breaking down a task into small, more manageable parts and putting them in order. Analyzing a task helps anyone learn what's involved in a task and teach it to someone else. For example, think about how you go about brushing your teeth. How many skills are involved, and in what order would you place them?

Here's an example of a task analysis. Imagine brushing your teeth, a set of skills that you do automatically. Imagine now that you are going to teach this skill to someone who has lost their brushing habit or routine. With some thought, you could probably develop a list like the following:

Skill Name: Brushing My Teeth
Steps (in order):

1. Set out toothbrush, toothpaste, and floss.

2. Put toothpaste on brush.

3. Run water over toothbrush to wet it.

4. With an up-and-down motion, brush the upper teeth and then lower teeth. Take two minutes.

5. Rinse mouth.

Chapter 4: Thinking in New Ways
Strategies and Tools for Learning Six Thinking Skills

6. Rinse toothbrush and return it to its usual place.

7. Floss. (You may need to write a separate task analysis for flossing.

8. Put used floss in garbage.

Habit is a cable; we spin a thread of it every day and at last we cannot break it.

ANONYMOUS

Naming the skill and listing the steps or sub-skills for brushing your teeth is a task analysis. The strategy behind this step-by-step analysis is to give the person with a brain injury a chance to practice each part successfully before trying to do the whole task. You can use task analysis for helping your loved one relearn or practice any skill. Your needs and the needs of your loved one will be different from anyone else's. You will want to develop your own task analysis for each skill you and your loved one need to work on.

The task-analysis worksheet displayed on the next page will help you understand how you go about analyzing a task. After you have worked through this worksheet, look at the exercises and information sheets designed for the person with brain injury. Then you can teach this valuable cognitive skill to your loved one.

Now is a good time to pause and do this worksheet:

- (4-3) Task-Analysis Worksheet

You can use a worksheet like this for analyzing any task — life skills, communication skills, and any other skills you or your loved one need to learn. After you have done this worksheet, you will be better prepared to teach this valuable cognitive skill to your loved one.

After Brain Injury: Tools for Living
A Step-by-Step Guide for Caregivers and Survivors

Task-Analysis Worksheet

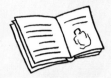

1. Name the overall task you want to examine:
   _____

2. Think about all the parts of this task and write them down. Don't worry about which step goes first, or next. Just write them down in the order you think of them.

   _____   _____
   _____   _____
   _____   _____
   _____   _____
   _____   _____
   _____   _____

3. Now put all the steps in order, starting from the first step and ending with the last step you will take to complete the task.

   Step #   Task or Step Required (in logical, chronological order)
   1   _____
   2   _____
   3   _____
   4   _____
   5   _____
   6   _____
   7   _____
   8   _____
   9   _____
   10 _____
   11 _____
   12 _____

Chapter 4: Thinking in New Ways
Strategies and Tools for Learning Six Thinking Skills

4. Try to do the task by following the steps you have written down. Have you missed some steps? Are all the steps in order? You will probably have to make some changes to your list. You may have to repeat this process several times until you have all the steps involved in the task you want to do.

5. Look carefully at each step. Do you have any learning aids that could act as cues, or are the words enough of a guide?

6. Write out the steps again below, including any changes you need to make. You now have finished making an instructional guide that you can use to help yourself or your loved one learn something new.

Step #   Task or Step Required (in logical, chronological order)

1 _____
2 _____
3 _____
4 _____
5 _____
6 _____
7 _____
8 _____
9 _____
10 _____
11 _____
12 _____

(4) Solving problems

Life presents everyone with many problems every day, and sometimes the problems seem endless. The person with a brain injury is constantly being challenged to solve problems like these:

- How do I clean up this mess?

- I feel overwhelmed! What do I need to do?

- I've run out of money, but not out of month. How will I manage?

One strategy for problem-solving is to give the person with a brain injury a model for learning or relearning this important cognitive skill. A model gives steps to follow every time a problem needs to be solved. One helpful model uses the letters in the word "PROBLEMS" as a way of remembering the steps to follow to solve problems:

P = State the **problem** you're having or put it in writing.

R = List the **reasons** you might be having this problem. Think of as many reasons or causes as you can.

O = **Organize** the possible reasons from most to least probable.

B = **Build** your confidence by building in some positive new ways of seeing the problem. Ask for feedback.

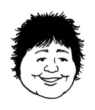

Lynne says . . . Because these skills are so basic to effective life management, we also include them in our TOM Binder System, which is contained in a separate binder. Please see ordering information at the back of this book.

Chapter 4: Thinking in New Ways
Strategies and Tools for Learning Six Thinking Skills

For example, after asking your friend for feedback, you might be able to say, "Jane says I'm on the right track."

Smile...it makes others wonder what you're thinking.

ANONYMOUS

L = **Locate** your personal power now. Come up with some solutions that address the problem and its cause. Pick the top three solutions.

E = **Evaluate** your solutions, then pick the top one. It may be enough to solve the problem.

M = **Make** a decision. Write down what you will do first, then next, and next again, to try out the solution to your problem.

S = **Start** solving your problem.

This model uses the word PROBLEMS as an acronym, a combination of letters that stands for a larger meaning. With practice, you and your loved one will memorize this acronym and what it stands for, and be able to apply it to any problem.

On the following page, look for this worksheet:

- (4-4) Problem-Solving Worksheet

Now is a good time to pause and do this worksheet. After you have done this worksheet, you will be better prepared to teach this valuable cognitive skill to your loved one.

After Brain Injury: Tools for Living
A Step-by-Step Guide for Caregivers and Survivors

W 4-4

Problem-Solving Worksheet

Use the letters of the word PROBLEMS as steps to follow when you go about solving a problem.

P State the problem you are facing at this time:
_____
_____

R Review why you might be having this problem right now.
Think of four possible reasons:
1. _____
2. _____
3. _____
4. _____

O Organize your list of possible reasons in order from MOST to LEAST likely:
Most likely: Reason # _____
Quite likely: Reason # _____
Not very likely: Reason # _____
Least likely: Reason # _____

B Build your confidence in how you see the problem. Ask someone else for feedback on the three sections you have just filled in.
Who will you ask? _____
After you ask, how would you summarize the person's feedback?
_____
_____

L Locate your personal power now. What solutions would start solving the problem and dealing with the reasons you are having the problem?
List three solutions:
1. _____
2. _____
3. _____

E Evaluate the solutions you just listed. Look carefully at them. Pick the most likely solution to your problem and state it here:
_____

M Make a decision. Decide what you will do to solve the problem.
First, I'll _____
And then, I'll _____

S Start solving your problem!

Chapter 4: Thinking in New Ways
Strategies and Tools for Learning Six Thinking Skills

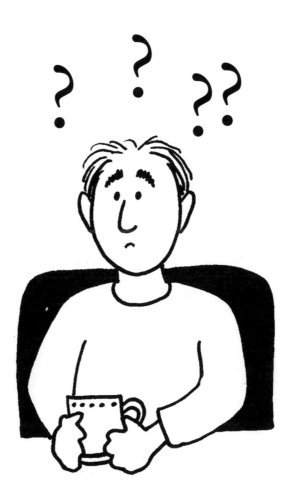

Q: What if the solution to my problem has many steps?

A: Any multi-step set of related activities that take place over time is called a project in this book. See the next page for help in planning projects.

(5) Planning projects

If all else fails, read the directions.

ANONYMOUS

A project is any activity that takes place over time, needs planning, and involves several steps and goals. Some projects take place every day. Others happen once in a while or maybe just once a year. However often they happen, projects involve activities that contain many steps. Here are some examples: paying bills, cleaning the refrigerator, filing papers, putting photos into albums, returning phone calls, answering e-mails, making appointments, doing exercises, or planning a holiday.

Making an informed decision may not be a project if you can complete it all in one time period and do not need to make that decision again. For example, taking your dog for a walk may not be a project if it involves tasks that you do not need to plan. In this case it would be considered an activity, not a project.

The strategy for helping a person with a brain injury plan a project is to break the project down into a logical, step-by-step process that gradually answers these questions:

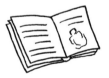

- What is the project needing to be done?
- What is the goal of the project?
- Why is the project important to you?
- What steps are involved in achieving the goal of the project?
- Who will do each step?
- When will each step probably be completed?
- When was each step actually completed?
- When was the project finished?

There are just a few steps involved in planning a project. First, for each new project, start a new project sheet like the one you see on the following page. On the new project sheet, write in the project's goal. For example: "Pay the bills on time."

Write down why this goal is important for you. For example, you might write, "I want to stop feeling guilty about my unpaid bills." Think about the steps you need to take to achieve this goal.

Write each step down in the order that you need to do it to achieve the goal. List just one step or task at a time.

Step #	Task or Activity Needing to be Done	Assigned To?	Date Due:	Done?
1.	Decide on a day each week to pay bills	Me	Tuesday	✔

In the box at the bottom left of the project sheet, draw a picture to remind you about your goal. If you have other projects related to this one, list them in the box located at the bottom right of the project sheet.

Now is a good time to pause and do the worksheet on the following page:

- (4-5) Project-Planning Worksheet

After you have done this worksheet, you will be better prepared to teach this valuable cognitive skill to your loved one.

After Brain Injury: Tools for Living
A Step-by-Step Guide for Caregivers and Survivors

W 4–5

Project-Planning Worksheet

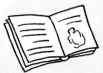

Project #_____

My project's goal: _____

Why this goal is important to me: _____
_____

Steps needed to achieve this goal, in order from first to last:

Step #	Task or Activity Needing to be Done	Assigned To?	Date Due:	Done?

Place picture cue here.

Related Project #	Project Goal	Done?

(6) Managing time

Another important skill for recovery is being able to organize and manage your time and activities. When you say someone is organized, you probably mean that person appears to be managing time, activities, and commitments in a logical or systematic way.

Many people with brain injuries say that they do not have time and energy to do all they need to do. Managing time does not only affect people with brain injury. You might find this a skill you need to learn, too, with all the tasks involved in your life as a caregiver. Time management becomes an essential activity for bringing balance back into your life and your loved one's.

A strategy that many caregivers and survivors find very helpful for managing time is setting aside daily time for planned activities. One of the easiest ways to do this is by creating a weekly time and activity calendar. All the information you need is right on each block of the calendar.

On the following page, you will see a sample calendar:

- (4-6) Weekly Time and Activity Calendar

Here are some important things to remember when using this calendar:

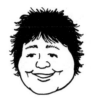

- Divide each day of the week into two sections.

- In the top section, put your regular commitments and

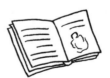

Lynne says... Through experience, we have found that effective time and activity management involve project-planning. You can find Project-Planning worksheets at the back of this book and in the TOM Binder System.

After Brain Injury: Tools for Living
A Step-by-Step Guide for Caregivers and Survivors

W 4-6

Weekly Time and Activity Calendar

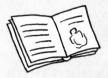

Weekly Time and Activity Calendar Month of: _____

Things I do every day, every week:

Time / Day & Date	Date: Monday	Date: Tuesday	Date: Wednesday	Date: Thursday	Date: Friday	Date: Sat/Sun
Morning						
Afternoon						
Evening						

Things I do only sometimes, such as calls and special projects:

Calls O = Outgoing I = Incoming						
Projects (special ones that don't happen regularly)						
Other						

Chapter 4: Thinking in New Ways
Strategies and Tools for Learning Six Thinking Skills

the things you do daily, every week, in three time blocks: morning, afternoon, and evening.

- In the bottom section, put things you do only sometimes, but need or expect to do this week, such as phone calls, appointments, visiting, fun activities, and special projects you want to work on.

If it takes a lot of words to say what you have in mind, give it more thought.

DENNIS ROCH

To start, place only one activity or project per block for your loved one. Otherwise, she/he is likely to become exhausted. Later you can place more than one project or activity in each daily time block.

Make up codes for certain kinds of activities or projects. That way, the calendar doesn't become too crowded with words. For example, you could make up codes for two kinds of telephone calls. **I** could stand for Incoming, calls you expect to receive. **O** could stand for Outgoing, calls you plan to make.

Use the codes to plan your calls and remember the commitments of others to call you. If you need a more detailed reminder, buy a phone-message book that supplies you with space to write in why the call happened and what you are still awaiting as a result. For example, you want to remember to call your friend Paul about a weekend trip. Enter: "Paul – trip (O) 604-732-0001" For example, a helper has promised to phone you with an appointment time. Enter: "physio – appointment (I) 604-224-5108" When calls are incomplete, move them to the next day's CALLS section.

Big Ideas are so hard to recognize, so fragile, so easy to kill. Don't forget that, all of you who don't have them.

JOHN ELLIOT, JR.

Once you have more energy, make a second, portable calendar that you can take with you to work or to other activities. Every week, start a new calendar. If you are using two calendars, make sure you coordinate them. Keep past calendars in a file called Weekly Calendars in case you have to look up something later.

A separate phone-message book also works for keeping everyone on track with projects. If you are helping your loved one, write down her/his task on a phone-message pad that creates an extra copy. Your loved one's copy stays in the book. You take the front copy and keep it as a reminder of the task.

With this calendar and all the other strategies and tools described in this chapter, you can help your loved one learn and practice important thinking skills. You too will benefit. Now you are ready to look at helping your loved one change behavior, which is often affected by injury to the brain. That's the topic of the final chapter of this book.

5 Changing Behavior

Learning goals for this chapter

This chapter focuses on changing behavior that has been affected by the physical and psychological trauma of brain injury. First the chapter looks briefly at what works when changing behavior. Then the chapter looks at stages most people go through in learning new behaviors. By becoming aware of these stages, you will start to understand why people with brain injuries find it hard to make changes in behavior last a long time.

The main part of this chapter presents three models for changing behavior. These models will help you understand what makes changes in behavior possible, what makes changes in behavior happen, and how to decide what changes are needed.

In this chapter, you will have a chance to:

- see that behavior happens in stages
- look at the principles behind changing behavior
- learn three models for changing behavior
- use the models to help a person with brain injury change behavior
- work through an example of how to change anger as a problem behavior

Introduction

Start by doing the necessary, then the possible and suddenly you are doing the impossible.

St. Francis of Assisi

The other chapters in this book have talked about the kinds of changes that have happened to your loved one and to you as a caregiver after brain injury. Both the trauma and the recovery process have changed you both.

Some changes came about as a result of the trauma that you, your loved one, and your family and friends experienced when the brain injury happened. For example, you made changes in your life in order to become a caregiver for your loved one.

Other changes happened as you and your loved one started to recover psychologically from the trauma. While reading this book, you have learned ways of becoming more self-aware and recovering emotionally. You have also learned about strategies and tools for thinking in new ways. You have started using these ideas, strategies, and tools to help your loved one in his/her recovery. You are ready to start working on changing behavior that came about as a result of the trauma of brain injury.

Like Chapter 4, this chapter looks at something that you, as a caregiver, might not think you have experienced yourself. However, it's likely that your behavior has been affected by the trauma of the brain injury to your loved one and everything that has happened since then. This chapter will increase your understanding of behavior and show you ways to help your loved one. In the process, you can use this knowledge for changing some of your own behavior.

What is behavior?

Behavior is an act or expression that others can easily see. Even though it never shows the whole picture, most behavior says something about how a person feels and thinks.

When you are trying to change, behavior is easier to measure than thoughts or feelings. When you set goals, changes in behavior are easier to see than changes in thoughts or feelings. That's why looking at behavior is an important part of recovery.

> Behavior = an act or expression that others can easily see.

Why change behavior?

As a caregiver, you know that an injury to the brain can cause a variety of behaviors. After the brain injury happened, your loved one might have started behaving in ways you had never seen before. Some of these new behaviors lasted only a short while. Others have lasted a long time.

Some of the changes were easy for you to get used to. Others are hard for you and your loved one to deal with. You might have some behaviors of your own that are hard for you and your loved one to deal with. That's why this chapter is looking at ways of changing behavior.

What Works When Changing Behavior

Mike says... If you have bought the separate Pocket Guide, you will have a pocket-sized set of cue cards for all the ideas you see here about changing behavior. With pictures and words, these cue cards give you a visual way of reminding your loved one about behavior you have worked on. You and your loved one will find these cards very helpful.

Many people have studied ways of changing behavior and have figured out what works best. The list ranges from identifying what you wish to change to finding a way to keep track of your new behavior:

- Start by identifying carefully what you wish to change. Be as specific as possible. For example, instead of saying, "I want to stop being angry," try saying, "I want to change my angry reactions to other drivers when I'm in a car."

- Set realistic and achievable goals for change. To increase your chances of success, work on your large goals step by step, one small goal at a time. To use the above example, you might start by saying, "I want to drive to the grocery store and back without feeling angry at other drivers."

- Decide how to measure your new behavior. Most people measure new behavior in two ways: how often it happens and how long it lasts when it happens. To use the above example, you might say, "When I drive to the grocery store today, I will count each time I feel impatient but don't get angry."

- Find a way to keep track of your new behavior. Buy a journal to write in or make a chart that you can fill in every day. To use the above example, you might say, "I'll keep this chart handy in the car."

- Show an attitude of willingness toward learning new things and changing. To use the above example, you might say, "I saw a book on how to manage anger. I'm going to read it. Maybe it will have some ideas that can help me."

Helping Your Survivor

Daily Reminders

For everyone, changing behavior is an ongoing process. It requires care and attention over time. We all sometimes need reminders that we have learned new behaviors. This is particularly true for the person with a brain injury.

To teach a survivor new behaviors:

1. Present the new behavior.

2. Practice the new behavior.

3. Remind with gentle and positive encouragement.

At times, the new behavior you have both worked hard to achieve may seem to disappear. Expect this. Don't panic.

Be prepared to remind your loved one about the appropriate new behavior — again and again. The reminders will become part of your everyday life together. Over time, she/he will need your reminders less and less. The new behavior will become part of your loved one's long-term memory.

Anger opens the mouth and shuts the mind.

ANONYMOUS

Two final things that work when changing behavior are positive self-talk and rewarding yourself often for your progress. An example of positive self-talk might be: "Good for me! Last week I would have honked my horn at that driver. I still felt angry, but my anger didn't last long." An example of rewarding yourself might be: "Today when I reached the store without feeling angry once, I sat down and took five minutes for a cup of tea. That's a treat for me, and it helped me stay relaxed."

Stages in Learning New Behavior

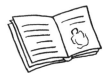

Changing behavior requires learning, and learning takes place in a series of stages, each stage leading to the next. Here are the five basic stages most people go through while learning a new behavior:

1. **Acquisition**. The teacher gives the learner new information. The learner receives new information.

2. **Rehearsal**. The teacher and the learner practice the skill in a safe environment. A safe environment is a place where the teacher and the learner can take the time they need to practice the skill and make mistakes without anyone else judging them. This safe environment will be different for everyone.

3. **Practice**. The learner tries out the new behavior in the "real" world.

4. **Integration**. After constant practice, the learned new skill becomes a habit that can be taken for granted.

5. **Sharing**. The learner shares the new skill with others and may even help them learn the skill. The learner becomes a teacher.

Remember what the previous section said about taking small, achievable steps when changing behavior? Taking small, achievable steps works particularly well for a person with a brain injury, with success built into each step.

That means you as the caregiver need to begin with the attitude of being open to partial outcomes. What are partial outcomes? They are the small successes, the tiny bits of change made as the person works on a larger goal. You can look on partial outcomes as success. Even the tiniest change is enough. Why? Because with practice and reminders, more change will happen.

For example, you and your loved one might be working on changing a certain behavior. Maybe your loved one, when feeling happy and sociable, jabs you hard on the arm. Your big goal might be that your loved one just smile when feeling happy and sociable, and not feel the need to jab you. A partial outcome might be that your loved one, when feeling happy and sociable, taps you on the arm instead of jabbing you.

Learning that takes place between a caregiver and a person with brain injury is a bit different from an ordinary teacher-student situation. You might find your loved one more

Lynne says... This is probably the most important thing to remember about changing behavior in people with brain injuries: For your loved one, even partial success can result in a move toward greater independence, self-confidence, and development of skills. And that means life can be easier and more comfortable for everyone.

Behavior is a mirror in which everyone shows his image.

GOETHE

open to your help if you take the role of a guider rather than a teacher. You could also let your loved one know that sometimes you are a learner, too. Sometimes your loved one can take the role of the guider/teacher.

Once you have gone through all five stages of learning a new behavior, from Acquisition to Sharing, your new behavior becomes a consistent, permanent part of how you are. You don't have to think about it — it's there every time you need it. However, Stages 4 and 5 of learning (Integration and Sharing) require a high level of self-awareness. That's why many people with brain injuries find it hard to make new behaviors last. Your loved one might not have enough self-awareness to reach the fourth and fifth stages of learning. This may change as your loved one recovers, but it may not.

By now, you might have some questions about how to start changing behavior. The next section presents models for changing behavior.

Three Models for Changing Behavior

In this section, you will see three models for changing behavior. A model gives steps to follow every time a problem needs to be solved. Each of these models shows a different way of understanding and changing behavior. Together, they give you several ways of working with your loved one: Mastery Model, Five-Stage Model, and Task-Analysis Model.

Mastery Model

Because it focuses on readiness, skills building, and confidence, the Mastery Model applies only to the first three stages of learning: Acquisition, Rehearsal, and Practice.

The Mastery Model shows that in order to learn something, you must have the following:

- readiness to learn the new skill

- knowledge of the skills involved in the new skill

- confidence to express or perform the new skill

This explains why sometimes you might have trouble learning or teaching something. The learner, whether that's you or your loved one, might not have the skills and confidence to feel ready to learn.

The Mastery Model

Readiness
+ Skills Building
+ Confidence
───────────────
= Mastery

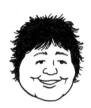

Lynne says... It's important to remember that whatever model you use to help change your loved one's behavior, the methods are focused on specific goals. These methods have been used by many people and will work to bring growth and progress. They will not make changes that last forever. Forever is not our goal. Providing skills and encouraging confidence are our goals.

Readiness is not a skill, but a part of normal development. You will understand the concept of developmental readiness if you think about the fact that most babies need to balance enough to sit up before they can crawl, and crawl before they start to walk. The physical and psychological development that takes place during the crawling and sitting stage is necessary for learning to walk. This developmental progression, step by step by step, is the same for other types of learning.

In other words, when you are not physically and psychologically ready to do something, no amount of skills-building and confidence-boosting will help. When you are ready to learn, you will begin learning and will likely find it much easier to learn. Once you have readiness to learn, you are ready to see what skills you already have to contribute to the new behavior and start to build up your confidence.

Five-Stage Goal-Setting Model

Once you are ready to change behavior, the Five-Stage Goal-Setting Model gives you an easy-to-follow method for bringing about the change.

Stage 1 – Set Your Goal

For you or your loved one, it's the same: Your goal must be personal. Work only on goals that you want, not what others choose for you. Think only about behavior you really want to change. You might find it helpful to look again at the (4-1) Clear Goal-Setting worksheet in Chapter 4. You will also find the worksheet on the following page helpful:

- (5-1) Setting Your Hazy Goal

W 5-1

Chapter 5: Changing Behavior
Three Models for Changing Behavior

Setting Your Hazy Goal Worksheet

Goals can be as big or as small as you need them to be. They can cover a wide range of human behavior.

1. Write down your Hazy Goal. A Hazy Goal is a vague sense of something that you want — something you hope for. In this case, choose a Hazy Goal for a behavior you want to change. Don't worry about how your goal sounds to someone else. Make sure that it is your Hazy Goal, not someone else's goal for you.

   _____
   _____
   _____
   _____

2. Look at your Hazy Goal, then look at the following list. Think about what kind of goal your goal is and put a checkmark beside it.

   ❏ personal growth or recovery (which will also change my behavior)
   ❏ thinking or cognitive (my thinking does affect my behavior)
   ❏ behavior (something others can see)
   ❏ impulse control (if you or your loved one has a "short fuse")

3. Now, think about why your Hazy Goal is important to you. If you are not clear about your reasons for changing your behavior, you might end up just trying to change to please others. It might help to check off one or more of the following reasons why your Hazy Goal is important to you.

   ❏ I will feel better for accomplishing it.
   ❏ I need to achieve this goal as part of a larger dream that I have.
   ❏ I am suffering the effects of not reaching this goal.
   ❏ This goal reflects an important value that I hold. Here's how I describe this value: _____

   Other reasons:
   _____
   _____
   _____

Stage 2 – Identify What Needs to Be Done

Clearly identify what needs to be done in order to accomplish the goal one step at a time. Is each step so clear that you would know when you are successful? Would anyone else watching you know when you complete a step?

Do a clarity check:

If time is important, how have you included it in your goal?
_____
_____

If you saw someone else doing this behavior, how would you recognize it? _____
_____

How would anyone watching you know for sure when you are doing the changed behavior? _____
_____

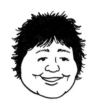

Lynne says . . . Read each stage on your own first. Give yourself some time to think about the ideas presented in this chapter before you try to teach them to your loved one.

Stage 3 – Measure Change in Behavior

It must be easy for you to measure your changes in behavior. Otherwise, you will stop measuring or give up the new behavior. There are two ways to measure behavior:

- measuring how often a behavior occurs (also referred to as frequency measurement)

- measuring how long a behavior lasts when it happens (also referred to as interval measurement)

Chapter 5: Changing Behavior
Three Models for Changing Behavior

Since you will be changing your behavior at the same time as you are doing other things in your everyday life, you need a simple method of measurement. A graph gives you a quick and easy way of tracking your behavior or your loved one's. On the following page you will see a sample of this worksheet:

Action may not always be happiness, but there is no happiness without action.

ANONYMOUS

- (5-2) Using a Graph to Measure Behavior Worksheet

There is a copy of the worksheet in the Resources setion of the book. On the sample, write down in the Goal Title box what behavior you are focusing on at this time. Then follow these steps:

1. Write down your Hazy Goal below and the first step you can take to achieve that goal.

   My Hazy Goal:_____

   My first action step: _____
   _____

2. Do you have a time goal with this step? If so, put the date that you expect to have achieved this first step here:
   _____

3. Look at your first step. Choose which method will be easiest for you to count daily:

   ❏ I will count how many times I do this behavior daily (frequency counting). Try to find a way to use frequency counting. It is simpler than interval counting.

After Brain Injury: Tools for Living
A Step-by-Step Guide for Caregivers and Survivors

W 5-2

Using a Graph to Measure Behavior Worksheet

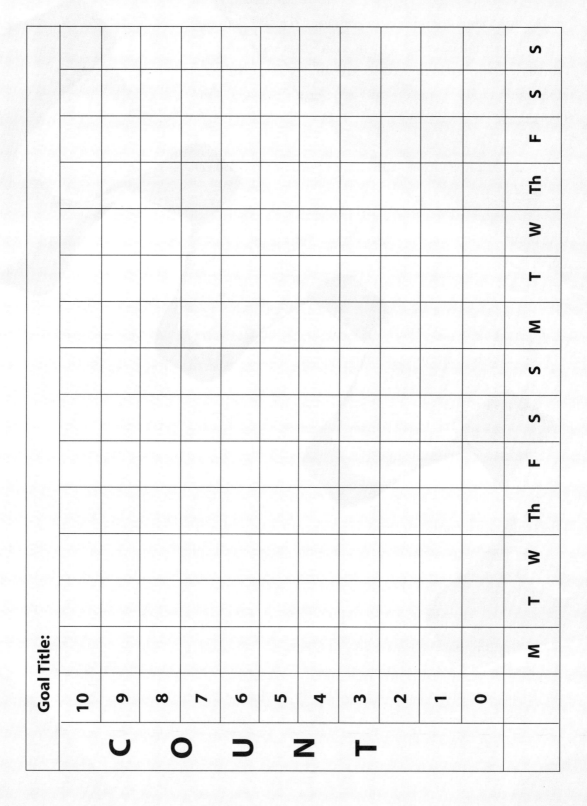

Chapter 5: Changing Behavior
Three Models for Changing Behavior

❏ I will count how much time I spend doing this behavior daily (interval counting).

4. If you have decided to use frequency counting (the easiest way to measure your behavior), you need to choose what you will use as "counters." Many people choose small, light items such as pennies or popcorn kernels. You probably can think of other items you can use.

5. Start counting and measuring your behavior:

- Each morning, at the beginning of your day, put your counters in your left pocket.

- Every time you do the behavior that you are focusing on, move a counter to your right pocket.

- At the end of the day, count the counters in your right pocket. Enter that amount on the correct day on the graph paper.

- Move all the day's counters to a place where you will see them the next morning, as you dress.

- Use the graph paper to record your daily counts.

- Track and graph your behavior for at least one week.

- At the end of each week, connect the graphed points.

6. If you choose interval counting, you will need a timer that can add up total time. In a journal, record the

Lynne says … Whether you have a brain injury or whether you just want change, you need to be able to measure your progress toward your goals.

Goals are dreams with deadlines.

<small>ANONYMOUS</small>

behavior each time it happens and for how long. Then add up the times at the end of the day.

7. After one week, use the information on the graph to set a new goal or action step. For example, you might decide to increase the number of times that the new behavior happens.

Stage 4 – Keep Track of Your Progress

Some goals require just one or two steps to achieve. For these goals, you see progress quickly. Other goals are more complicated, with many steps. You might not have known all the steps involved when you started. For these goals, it's harder to tell how you're progressing, and it's important to keep track of your progress.

By now, you are already using a graph to count the number of times you do your new behavior every week. Once you have kept graphs for several weeks, you will have the information that you need for regular reviews. The worksheet on the following page shows you how to do a review:

- (5-3) Evaluating Progress Toward My Goal Worksheet

Stage 5 – Reward and Celebrate Achievement

For you and your loved one, achieving your goals can be both hard work and a reason to celebrate. While you are changing your behavior, take time to celebrate even the little accomplishments and successes. This has an important purpose: It encourages you both to hope for more. Once you hope for more, you start to create even more dreams…and goals…and successes. And on it goes.

W 5-3

Chapter 5: Changing Behavior
Three Models for Changing Behavior

Evaluating Progress Toward My Goal Worksheet

1. My achievable, realistic, measurable goal is: _____
   _____

2. The behavior I am counting and keeping track of at this time is:
   _____

3. Once you have kept track of your progress for several weeks on graphs, make a chart comparing your weekly goal (frequency or interval) to your actual counts (the number of counters you moved in a week).

	Week 1	Week 2	Week 3	Week 4	Week 5
My weekly goal					
My actual count					

4. Look at the chart. Decide whether your progress is:

   ❏ On track. You will keep on doing what is working.
   ❏ Off track. You need to make a change in your goal or in the behavior you're working on.

5. Decide what change to make.

   ❏ Be more realistic. Break this behavior into smaller pieces and then count for the next week.
   ❏ Keep the step, but be kinder to yourself. Try lowering your weekly goal so that you just have to stretch a little to succeed.
   ❏ Ask for help about how to re-shape your goal or your behavior.

6. Plan the changes you need to make. For this, you can use a project-planning worksheet. For ideas, see the Project-Planning Worksheet in Chapter 4.

If you always do what you always did, you'll always get what you always got.

ANONYMOUS

It helps to make a list of the rewards you like. Include big rewards and little ones. Keep your list handy so that you can easily see how to reward yourself often. Here are some ideas other people have:

- taking a break

- making time to visit a friend

- having a cup of tea and watching the clouds go by

- creating realistic and positive affirmations that fit you

- accepting that "I worked hard on this project and didn't give up"

- recognizing that "I expressed my displeasure in a respectful way"

- having time for fun

- patting yourself on the back

You can use this worksheet on the next page to list your own ideas or those of your loved one:

- (5-4) Rewarding/Celebrating Achievement Worksheet

Rewarding/Celebrating Achievement Worksheet

Make a list of the rewards and celebrations you would like as you achieve your goals.

_____

_____

_____

_____

_____

_____

_____

_____

_____

_____

_____

_____

What if you can't describe the change you want? Sometimes it is easier to see behavior that is a problem, but not nearly as easy to see what the change ought to be. For example, you might find yourself saying often, "Stop doing that" when you see your loved one behave in a rude or offensive way. It's harder to decide what positive behavior you hope to see instead. You need a method of turning your desire for change into reality one step at a time. The Task-Analysis Model gives you that method.

Task-Analysis Model

In Chapter 4, you saw that analyzing a task is one strategy for learning or relearning thinking skills. By doing the Task-Analysis Worksheet in that chapter, you found that analyzing a task involves breaking it down into small, more manageable parts and putting them in order.

The Task-Analysis Model is based on this idea — that large or difficult skills can be broken down into smaller skills or steps, each one completed before the next one is started. This breaking down makes it much easier to understand and learn all the skills required for a goal.

To perform a task analysis, you need only watch someone doing the desired behavior. Stop watching the undesirable behavior for a moment and watch a star performer of the desired behavior. For example, maybe your loved one needs to learn how to act as if she/he is listening to others. You have probably tried saying, "Stop interrupting" and found that doesn't give your loved one enough information about what to change.

> Watch a star performer of the desired behavior.

Chapter 5: Changing Behavior
Three Models for Changing Behavior

If you use the Task-Analysis Model, you find someone you think is a good listener and you observe that person. You will probably see that a good listener does much more than simply not interrupt. A good listener might also use other techniques for active listening, such as:

- smiling and looking directly at the speaker

- nodding and encouraging the speaker to go on

- restating what the speaker has said

- waiting for a few seconds after the speaker has finished

- taking a turn as a speaker only if the speaker is finished

Just from watching a good listener carefully and writing down all the steps that he/she does in listening, you are doing a task analysis. Extra worksheets follow in the Resources section.

After developing a task analysis, you then need to test it. How do you test it? Try doing each step of the behavior as you have written it out, or ask a friend to follow your task analysis. Can your friend follow the steps you have described, or have you left some out? Your loved one will need to see and practice every single step involved.

Only by testing your analysis can you become aware of any missing or incomplete steps. Steps that may be too large or complex will also become obvious. If you need to make big steps even smaller, divide each step into separate mini-steps.

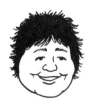

Lynne says . . . As you become comfortable with doing task analysis, it will become easier each time. Once you have learned how to do a task analysis, it is important to include your loved one.

Nobody plans to fail, they just fail to plan.

ANONYMOUS

Once you have made changes, test the task analysis again, to make sure you have included all the required steps. After you have finished the testing stage, you can start using your task analysis with your loved one. Congratulations! You have now developed your own instructional tool.

Task analysis is just one of the three models presented in this chapter. These three models will assist you as you make changes in your own behavior and in your loved one's behavior.

If you are not sure whether you or your loved one is ready for change, read over the information on the Mastery Model. Once you and your loved one feel ready for change, it is time to start step-by-step goal-setting using the Five Stage Goal-Setting Model.

Every once in a while, you will find that you can identify a problem, but not know the solution. When you can identify a problem and have willingness to change, but don't quite know how to teach the skill, try task analysis. Break skills into smaller component steps. Become a star observer. You will find your way to changing behavior.

An Example of Changing Behavior: Changing Anger

This final section gives you an example of how you can use the models in this chapter to start changing anger as your usual response to frustrating or difficult situations.

Anger is an emotion many caregivers and survivors express often after brain injury. Of course, there are times when anger is exactly the emotion that you need to bring about change. In the physical recovery stage, you and your loved one might have used the extra energy that comes with anger to get people's attention and make sure that your loved one received a particular treatment.

Now, however, you might find that you are using anger more than you want. Your loved one, too, might be showing anger often. After brain injury, many survivors feel and express a lot of anger, and it becomes their usual response to frustrating or difficult situations. Like with many caregivers, you might find your loved one's anger to be one of the biggest problems you have to deal with.

When does anger become a problem? Anger becomes a problem when:

- It happens too often.
- It is too intense or extreme for the situation.
- It lasts too long.
- It leads to physical action.
- It affects relationships in a negative way.

If you don't know where you are going, every road will get you nowhere.

HENRY KISSINGER

One way of starting to change anger as a problem behavior in you or your loved one could involve these steps:

- setting a goal
- identifying your anger style and trigger conditions
- measuring anger
- reviewing goals

Setting a weekly goal

Once you have identified anger in yourself or your loved one as a problem, you need to set a weekly goal for change. For example, you might want to reduce how often you feel angry when someone asks you about your loved one, feel angry less often, or you might want to stop your loved one's anger from leading to physical action. For setting a goal, you will find the Goal-Setting Worksheet shown earlier in this chapter helpful.

Identifying your anger style and trigger conditions

Identifying your anger style and trigger conditions are important first steps in changing anger as a behavior.

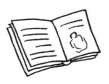

Anger style

Anger style is how you feel or express anger. Each person's style of feeling and expressing anger will be different. Yours will probably be different from your loved one's. You might see a style that describes you or your loved one in this list:

- I am a stuffer. I keep my anger inside me.
- I am a volcano. I explode when I feel angry.
- I am a pot on a hot stove. I simmer and boil constantly.
- I am a blamer. I usually blame others when I feel angry.
- I am a person who handles my anger well. I express myself assertively and show respect for others.

Chapter 5: Changing Behavior
An Example of Changing Behavior: Changing Anger

How would you describe your anger style and that of your loved one?

After all is said and done, more is said than done.

ANONYMOUS

Your anger style:
_____

Your loved one's anger style:
_____

Trigger conditions

Trigger conditions are situations where you or your loved one are very likely to react with anger. Again, each person's trigger conditions will be different. Here are some that many caregivers and survivors identify:

- **C**   Confusion (I feel lost and confused.)
- **R**   Reduced Stamina (I feel tired and overwhelmed.)
- **O**   Over-stimulation (I feel as if a thousand things are coming at me all at once.)
- **S**   Sad (I feel sad and have trouble seeing that things will get better.)
- **S**   Scared (I feel scared and worried.)

How would you describe your trigger conditions and those of your loved one?

Your trigger conditions:
_____
_____

Your loved one's trigger conditions:
_____
_____

Identifying trigger conditions

C Confusion (I feel lost and confused.)
R Reduced Stamina (I feel tired and overwhelmed.)
O Over-stimulation (I feel as if a thousand things are coming at me all at once.)
S Sad (I feel sad and have trouble seeing that things will get better.)
S Scared (I feel scared and worried.)

Measuring anger

As you have seen in this chapter, measurement is an important part of changing behavior, including anger as a problem behavior. Here is one method of measuring anger that you can use for yourself and your loved one:

- Count daily, using pennies or popcorn kernels. Start the day with some pennies or kernels in one pocket. Every time you feel angry, move a penny or kernel into another pocket.

- Make a graph. You will find the Using a Graph to Measure Behavior Worksheet shown earlier in this chapter helpful. Every evening, count the pennies or kernels you have moved from one pocket to another and write the total on the graph.

Chapter 5: Changing Behavior
An Example of Changing Behavior: Changing Anger

Reviewing goals

Once you have set a weekly goal and started identifying and measuring your anger, it is important to make a plan for regularly reviewing your goal. Show your graph once a week to someone you trust and talk about the results. Here are some things to talk about during your review:

- Decide whether you are on track with the goal you set.

- If you and your trusted person agree that you are on track, keep your weekly goal the same as last week. Your method of changing anger is working!

- If you both agree that you are not on track, do some problem-solving. You will find the Problem-Solving Worksheet in Chapter 4 helpful for this. You might need to change your goal or use another method of measuring behavior.

- Make copies of the worksheet on the following page and use it to make a plan for each new week:

(5-5) Weekly Goal Statement About Changing Anger

- Celebrate that you are starting to change anger as a problem behavior!

Not everything that counts can be counted, and not everything that can be counted counts.

Sign hanging in Albert Einstein's office at Princeton

After Brain Injury: Tools for Living
A Step-by-Step Guide for Caregivers and Survivors

W 5-5

Weekly Goal Statement About Changing Anger

Identify

The anger problem I am focusing on is:

_____

Describe

My goal meets all these conditions:

❏ important ❏ controllable
❏ conceivable ❏ measurable
❏ possible ❏ has no alternatives

Measure

The counters I'll use are:

_____(pennies or popcorn kernels)

Evaluate

The method of measurement I'll use is: *(check one)*
❏ frequency (how often) ❏ interval (how long)

My progress is: ❏ on track ❏ off track
The change I plan to make is:_____
_____

Reward

Review date:_____

I will celebrate my success by:_____
_____

Concluding Remarks

Lynne Mann

We have now come to the end of this book. It began as a practical project 25 years ago when community living was a new type of helping. Our work continues in the recognition that the time for involvement of professionals is relatively short, particularly in the community. The need to work collaboratively is obvious to most of us. This book has been my attempt to do that. As a psychologist, I believe that the best work is that which recognizes the complexity of both the human body and the human spirit. Simply seeing people as the sum total of their behavior and/or their thinking is clearly inadequate. We are so much more.

Emotional wellness, the processing of loss, and the growth of the indomitable human spirit are just as important parts of the human condition. We need to consider the complexity of life over and over in recovery. Appreciation of this complexity is what brings us into a far larger journey of belonging.

Mike Rossiter

The road to recovery goes on and on. Do not give up. Try the tools in this book. They work. Talk to others. Take care of yourself. Reach out for help every time you need it.

After Brain Injury: Tools for Living
A Step-by-Step Guide for Caregivers and Survivors

The Pocket Guide:
Key Points Related to Each Chapter

Throughout this book, you will see this icon. It refers to key points that will be summarized and included in **The Pocket Guide**. After reading the book you are holding, you may need only The Pocket Guide when helping your loved one. The Guide is meant as a compact reference tool for you, your survivor, and for other caregivers.

Chapter 1
- The best ways to know myself again
- The Psychological Self
- The Social Self
- The Real Self

Chapter 2
- How am I — right now?
- Self-based denial
- I am using a form of self-based denial when I …
- What can I do now to feel more safe?

Chapter 3
- Principles of emotional recovery
- Core issues in recovery
- What trauma roles look like
- Victim role
- Recovering from the victim role
- Rescuer role
- Recovering from the rescuer role
- Persecutor role
- Recovering from the persecutor role
- The five stages of emotional recovery
- Defining emotional recovery
- Willpower
- Willingness

Chapter 4
- What does thinking include?
- The frontal lobe of the brain
- To learn things more easily I should …
- The Mastery Model for learning
- Six elements of a good goal
- Five-Stage Goal-Setting Model
- Decision making
- Doing a task analysis
- Solving problems
- Planning projects
- Managing time

Chapter 5
- How do I change my behavior?
- Why do I measure my behavior?
- Measuring change in my behavior
- Identifying my anger style
- Identifying anger triggers
- Anger is a problem when …
- How can I deal with my impulsive outbursts?
- Weekly goal statement about changing anger
- More help is available …

Resources

Worksheets from all chapters

Further resources available

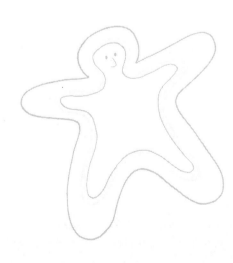

After Brain Injury: Tools for Living
A Step-by-Step Guide for Caregivers and Survivors

W 1–1

A Picture of My Psychological Self

Here is where you can draw a picture of your Psychological Self.

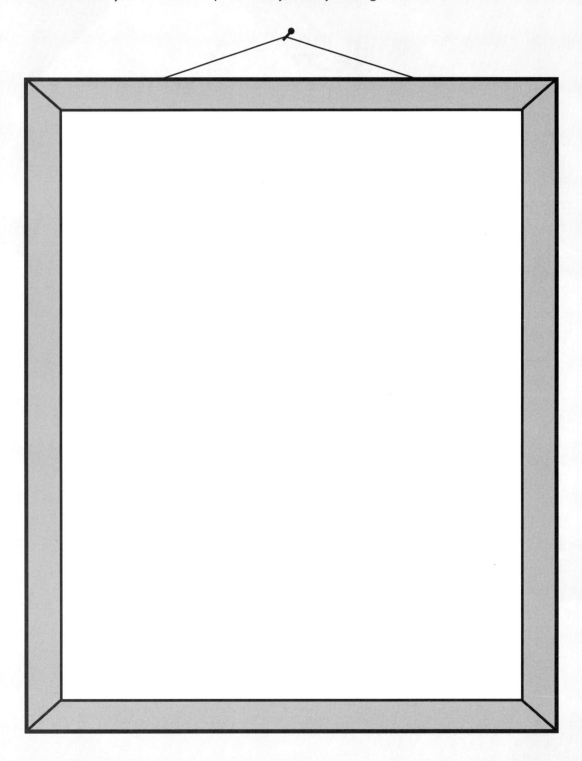

W 1-2

My Psychological Self Quiz

1. Imagine being in a social situation with strangers. You are alone, perhaps anxious. Your feelings of curiosity and pleasure are absent.

2. How would you act to protect yourself from feeling too much anxiety? *(Check one.)*

   ❏ become the party clown
   ❏ retreat to the yard outside where it is quiet
   ❏ take a deep breath, count to 5, and try to look interested

3. Whichever one you picked, decide if that behavior is an expression of *(Check one.)*

   ❏ your Social Self (whose job is to protect and communicate) OR
   ❏ your Real Self (whose jobs are to hold vulnerability, create and grow)

4. Decide which of the following are expressions of your Real Self (RS) and which are expressions of your Social Self (SS):

	Part of my Social Self	Part of my Real Self
Expressions:		
feeling a feeling	_____	_____
expressing a feeling	_____	_____
making an honest statement	_____	_____
wearing a mask	_____	_____
sharing a concern	_____	_____

   There are no right or wrong answers. What you will find is that the more you think about it, the more both parts of your Psychological Self are involved in many of your actions and feelings.

Confirm Your Understanding of the Psychological Self Worksheet

Part A

To have any conversation other than chit-chat, it helps to have a meaningful topic. Since we are talking about the Psychological Self, think of the most recent time you felt uncomfortable, just a little bit anxious. This will be the topic of conversation for your inner conversation.

Write a short description of what happened.
___

How did you feel? Name the feelings.
___

What thoughts did you have at the time?
___

What did you do and how did you express yourself?
___

W 1–3

Confirm Your Understanding of the Psychological Self Worksheet

Part B

Look at the Real Self/Social Self picture below and the information you wrote on the previous page. Decide whether each bit of information is a part of your Social Self talking or a part of your Real Self talking. Write each thought, feeling, action, need, desire, or impulse in the part of this drawing where you think it belongs.

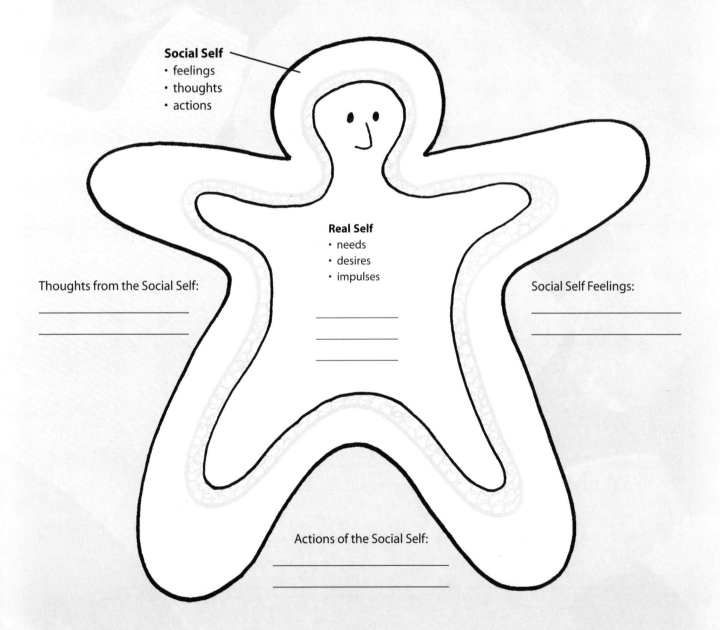

Social Self
- feelings
- thoughts
- actions

Real Self
- needs
- desires
- impulses

Thoughts from the Social Self:
_____
_____

Social Self Feelings:
_____
_____

Actions of the Social Self:
_____
_____

After Brain Injury: Tools for Living
A Step-by-Step Guide for Caregivers and Survivors

W 2-1

My Journal — A Blank Journal Page

Date _____ Time and Place _____

Topic _____

Social Self — thoughts and actions

_____
_____
_____
_____
_____
_____
_____
_____
_____
_____
_____
_____

Real Self — feelings, needs, desires, and impulses

_____
_____
_____
_____
_____
_____
_____
_____
_____
_____
_____

SST (Stop-Still-Think) Instructional Aid

After brain injury, thoughts, feelings, and actions can "jump out" without any planning. A person with a brain injury might have a "short fuse" or get angry too quickly or too much for a given situation. This is not a behavioral or an emotional problem. It is the result of disordered impulses. The person with a brain injury needs to re-learn how to control impulses.

Stop-Still-Think (SST) is a method for helping your loved one interrupt impulses, whether they are feelings, thoughts, or actions. The SST Aid consists of two sizes of cue cards.

SST stands for Stop, Still, Think.

Your goal is to use the SST aid to help your loved one train herself/himself to think of Stop-Still-Think every time she/he faces a situation needing help with impulse control. Both the large and small sets act as reminders to your loved one to stop, take a few breaths, and think before taking action. You can also use this tool for yourself.

Example of a Small SST Cue Card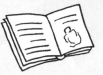

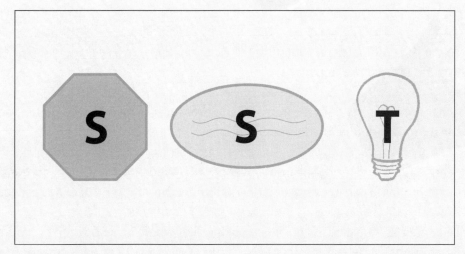

After Brain Injury: Tools for Living
A Step-by-Step Guide for Caregivers and Survivors

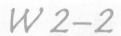

More About SST

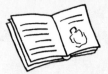

> As soon as you feel a twinge of a feeling or the beginning of a reactionary thought (a thought in reaction to another person's actions which affect you), follow the steps below.
>
> First, just for the moment, stop everything you are doing. If you are walking, STOP. If you are talking, STOP.
>
> Next, take some deep breaths. For just a few moments, focus only on this calming breathing. Use the wavy line to remind you of this inner calmness. Breathe your way there.
>
> Then, having stilled yourself, take another moment and ask yourself the following question: "Is there something I think or feel needs to be done now or should I hold my reaction inside me?"

SST can be used as a method for teaching systematic thinking to overcome impulsive thinking. SST replaces the Think-Do way of taking action impulsively with three steps — Stop, Still, Think — that happen before any action is taken. Placed in the wallet and throughout the home or at work, SST cue cards act as constant reminders of the three SST steps.

You will find a set of SST cue cards inserted into this book. The SST cue cards can be used in these ways:

- Place the large SST cards on your fridge so that your loved one sees them regularly until she/he has learned the steps.

- Attach them on the inside of the front door, to prompt your loved one to gather together all the things needed before leaving for the day.

- Tape an SST cue card inside the front cover of your loved one's daytimer or organizer, to remind him/her to carry out systematic, non-impulsive thoughts, feelings, or actions.

- Place a small SST cue card in your loved one's wallet where it can be seen every time the wallet is opened.

W 2-3

Exploring My Self-Based Denial Worksheet

Getting to know yourself again means looking at some of the ways in which you have protected yourself from loss, worry, and upheaval. Think of times when you used the kinds of denial shown in the chart below. Use the blank space to write a bit about your behavior. What caused it? What happened next? Another question you could ask yourself: "Do I still use this kind of denial often?"

Kinds of Self-Based Denial   **Description**

Regression   Reverting to an earlier, less adult way of acting (for example, stamping feet when angry).

Your personal example: _____
_____
_____

Wit & Humor   Using puns and other humor to distract yourself and others from uncomfortable feelings (for example, you act as the jokester, class clown, or party animal).

Your personal example: _____
_____
_____

Intellectualization   You use ideas and words to build a wall between you and your feelings. You talk only about ideas and words, not about feelings you might be having.

Your personal example: _____
_____
_____

After Brain Injury: Tools for Living
A Step-by-Step Guide for Caregivers and Survivors

Not Knowing When asked, you don't seem to know what you're feeling, thinking, or doing in the moment. Someone asks, "How are you?" and you answer, "I don't know." If the person tries to force you to answer, you immediately feel overwhelmed by all your worries and fears.

Your personal example: _____
_____
_____

Rationalization You try to explain your behavior with reasons that sound true, but aren't. For example, you arrive late for a meeting and say that the traffic slowed you down, when in fact you left home too late to allow for traffic slow-downs.

Your personal example: _____
_____
_____

Projection You blame others for your shortcomings. For example, you blame others for "making" you angry. You don't place responsibility for your anger where it belongs — with you.

Your personal example: _____
_____
_____

Reaction Formation You act opposite to the expected and usually you react with rage. For example, when hammering in a nail, you hit your thumb. You throw the hammer away angrily.

Your personal example: _____
_____
_____

W 3-2

Resources:
Worksheets

Identifying My Issues in Emotional Recovery

Below is a list of common core issues that people like you, who have experienced trauma, have identified. Look at the issues in the list below. Pick one issue that feels most relevant to you, today in this moment. Try not to think too much about which one you choose. There is no right or wrong answer.

Control	Healing denial through safety
Intimacy	Dealing with changed cognition
Courage and willingness to grow	Self-reliance
Emotional expression	Loss and grieving
Learning to trust again	Healing the self

1. Write the issue you have identified here: _____

2. Using the Five-Stage Emotional Recovery Model, identify your present stage of recovery for this issue:

   ❏ I am stuck, worried, and waiting. (Daily Survival stage)
   ❏ I have just re-identified this issue by naming it. While it may make me anxious, it feels exactly like the experience I am having. (Re-Identification stage)
   ❏ I am practicing a new response or behavior each time this issue happens. (Core Issues stage)
   ❏ While this issue was difficult to process, I am now a better...[problem-solver, person, negotiator]...because of facing it. (Integration stage)
   ❏ After working on recovery on this issue, I now know I have something to offer. I can contribute by...[volunteering, getting politically active, advocating]. (Genesis stage)

3. How will you keep track of your recovery work on this issue?

   ❏ I will journal daily and review my writing weekly.
   ❏ I will tell a friend about my journey in recovery.
   ❏ I will share my work with myself, tolerating change and the anxiety and hope it brings.
   ❏ I will review and redo this exercise weekly.

4. Your own ideas:
   ❏ _____
   ❏ _____

5. Decide on one action to do this week and write it here:
   _____
   _____

After Brain Injury, Tools for Living:
A Step-by-Step Guide for Caregivers and Survivors

Trauma Roles and Recovery Worksheet

Read the descriptions of the "I am…when I" trauma roles below and decide which role you take on most often. Put a checkmark beside each statement that is true for you. Then look at the "I can stop" list that follows. This list will give you examples of

I am in the victim role when I: *(Check any that are true for you.)*
- let other people do things for me and make plans for me
- believe that there is nothing I can do to change my own life
- don't believe I can get any of my needs met
- believe I am inferior to others and should step aside for them
- let other people make important decisions for me
- don't take responsibility for my own life
- avoid conflict and think I wouldn't get what I want anyway
- remain quiet about issues or feelings that are important to me
- expect others to hurt or disappoint me

I am rescuing when I: *(Check any that are true for you.)*
- do something I really don't want to do
- say "yes" when I mean "no"
- do something for someone even though that person is capable of doing it and should be doing it himself/herself
- meet people's needs without being asked and before I've agreed to do so
- do more than my fair share of work after my help is requested
- consistently give more than I receive in a particular situation
- fix other people's feelings
- do other people's thinking for them

I am persecuting when I: *(Check any that are true for you.)*
- tell other people what to do or give orders
- put other people down, make fun of them, or call people names
- invalidate other people's experiences
- manipulate others to get what I want
- control the behavior of others by threats or intimidation
- withhold my love and support from others as a way of punishing or intimidating them
- believe my own feelings and ideas are more important than anyone else's
- actively blame others for my own situation

what it would look like if you stopped taking on that particular role. Check off one thing on each list that you will start working on now.

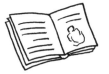

I can stop being a victim by: *(Check one that you will start working on now.)*
- ❏ educating myself on the difference between the victim role and the experience of victimization
- ❏ validating my own experiences, yet expanding my choices of how to respond to situations
- ❏ learning life skills such as assertiveness, communication and stress reduction
- ❏ seeking out people who will encourage a positive image of myself
- ❏ changing the circumstances that result in my feeling a victim
- ❏ breaking down my isolation

I can stop rescuing by: *(Check one that you will start working on now.)*
- ❏ limiting myself to doing no more than 50 per cent of the work in any relationship
- ❏ believing that others are not helpless
- ❏ giving others the information and support that can help them in changing their own lives
- ❏ being honest about my own feelings, needs and wants
- ❏ learning to separate my "need to be needed" from my genuine caring and compassion
- ❏ learning to set limits with others and to improve my feelings about myself
- ❏ identifying my own feelings, needs and wants

I can stop persecuting by: *(Check one that you will start working on now.)*
- ❏ learning to identify my feelings of anger
- ❏ finding suitable outlets for my feelings that are not hurtful to others
- ❏ using communication and assertion skills as an alternate way of communicating my thoughts and feelings
- ❏ learning to identify my feelings, needs, and wants
- ❏ working to feel better about myself
- ❏ remembering that it is my behavior that is the problem, not me or my feelings or needs

[The material on these two pages was written by a creative soul whose name could not be traced. Thanks!]

After Brain Injury: Tools for Living
A Step-by-Step Guide for Caregivers and Survivors

W 4–1

Clear Goal-Setting Worksheet

1. A Hazy Goal is a vague sense of something that you want — something you hope for. State your Hazy Goal:
   _____

2. Ask yourself whether your Hazy Goal is:

   ❏ personally important (Do I want to attain this goal?)
   ❏ achievable (Is this goal possible?)
   ❏ realistic (Can I do it?)
   ❏ measurable or countable (It must be, in order to work.)

   Then ask yourself: Does my Hazy Goal have alternatives, such as "Either I do this or I do that"? If so, choose one.

3. Does your Hazy Goal give you ways of measuring or counting your progress? How will you measure or count your progress?
   _____
   _____

4. What materials do you need for measuring your progress?
   _____
   _____

5. Describe the reward or celebration you plan when you succeed in reaching your goal.
   _____
   _____

6. Do you plan to achieve this goal by a certain time?
   No _____
   Yes, I plan to achieve this goal by _____ (insert the date here)

W 4-2

Resources:
Worksheets

Effective Decision-Making Worksheet

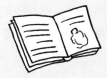

1. Think about the decision you are making. Write it down here:
   _____

2. List the other decisions you could make:

   A. I could _____

   OR
   B. I could _____

   OR
   C. I could _____

3. For each of the other decisions you could make, list the possible consequences, both negative and positive:

A.	B.	C.
positive consequences	positive consequences	positive consequences
_____	_____	_____
_____	_____	_____
negative consequences	negative consequences	negative consequences
_____	_____	_____
_____	_____	_____

4. Think carefully about the positive and negative consequences, then choose the best decision for you. Write down your best decision here:
   _____
   _____
   _____

After Brain Injury: Tools for Living
A Step-by-Step Guide for Caregivers and Survivors

W 4-3

Task-Analysis Worksheet

1. Name the overall task you want to examine:
   _____

2. Think about all the parts of this task and write them down. Don't worry about which step goes first, or next. Just write them down in the order you think of them.

   _____   _____
   _____   _____
   _____   _____
   _____   _____
   _____   _____
   _____   _____

3. Now put all the steps in order, starting from the first step and ending with the last step you will take to complete the task.

   Step #   Task or Step Required (in logical, chronological order)
   1   _____
   2   _____
   3   _____
   4   _____
   5   _____
   6   _____
   7   _____
   8   _____
   9   _____
   10   _____
   11   _____
   12   _____

Resources: Worksheets

4. Try to do the task by following the steps you have written down. Have you missed some steps? Are all the steps in order? You will probably have to make some changes to your list. You may have to repeat this process several times until you have all the steps involved in the task you want to do.

5. Look carefully at each step. Do you have any learning aids that could act as cues, or are the words enough of a guide?

6. Write out the steps again below, including any changes you need to make. You now have finished making an instructional guide that you can use to help yourself or your loved one learn something new.

Step # Task or Step Required (in logical, chronological order)

1. _____
2. _____
3. _____
4. _____
5. _____
6. _____
7. _____
8. _____
9. _____
10. _____
11. _____
12. _____

After Brain Injury: Tools for Living
A Step-by-Step Guide for Caregivers and Survivors

W 4-4

Problem-Solving Worksheet

Use the letters of the word PROBLEMS as steps to follow when you go about solving a problem.

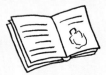

P State the problem you are facing at this time:
_____
_____

R Review why you might be having this problem right now.
Think of four possible reasons:
1. _____
2. _____
3. _____
4. _____

O Organize your list of possible reasons in order from MOST to LEAST likely:
Most likely: Reason # _____
Quite likely: Reason # _____
Not very likely: Reason # _____
Least likely: Reason # _____

B Build your confidence in how you see the problem. Ask someone else for feedback on the three sections you have just filled in.
Who will you ask? _____
After you ask, how would you summarize the person's feedback?
_____
_____

L Locate your personal power now. What solutions would start solving the problem and dealing with the reasons you are having the problem?
List three solutions:
1. _____
2. _____
3. _____

E Evaluate the solutions you just listed. Look carefully at them. Pick the most likely solution to your problem and state it here:
_____

M Make a decision. Decide what you will do to solve the problem.
First, I'll _____
And then, I'll _____

S Start solving your problem!

W 4–5

Resources:
Worksheets

Project-Planning Worksheet

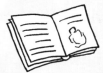

Project #_____

My project's goal: _____

Why this goal is important to me: _____
_____

Steps needed to achieve this goal, in order from first to last:

Step #	Task or Activity Needing to be Done	Assigned To?	Date Due:	Done?

Place picture cue here.

Related Project #	Project Goal	Done?

After Brain Injury: Tools for Living
A Step-by-Step Guide for Caregivers and Survivors

W 4-6

Weekly Time and Activity Calendar

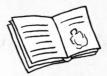

Weekly Time and Activity Calendar Month of: _____

Day & Date / Time	Date: Monday	Date: Tuesday	Date: Wednesday	Date: Thursday	Date: Friday	Date: Sat/Sun
Things I do every day, every week:						
Morning						
Afternoon						
Evening						
Things I do only sometimes, such as calls and special projects:						
Calls O = Outgoing I = Incoming						
Projects (special ones that don't happen regularly)						
Other						

W 5-1

Resources:
Worksheets

Setting Your Hazy Goal Worksheet

Goals can be as big or as small as you need them to be. They can cover a wide range of human behavior.

1. Write down your Hazy Goal. A Hazy Goal is a vague sense of something that you want — something you hope for. In this case, choose a Hazy Goal for a behavior you want to change. Don't worry about how your goal sounds to someone else. Make sure that it is your Hazy Goal, not someone else's goal for you.

   _____
   _____
   _____
   _____

2. Look at your Hazy Goal, then look at the following list. Think about what kind of goal your goal is and put a checkmark beside it.

   ❏ personal growth or recovery (which will also change my behavior)
   ❏ thinking or cognitive (my thinking does affect my behavior)
   ❏ behavior (something others can see)
   ❏ impulse control (if you or your loved one has a "short fuse")

3. Now, think about why your Hazy Goal is important to you. If you are not clear about your reasons for changing your behavior, you might end up just trying to change to please others. It might help to check off one or more of the following reasons why your Hazy Goal is important to you.

   ❏ I will feel better for accomplishing it.
   ❏ I need to achieve this goal as part of a larger dream that I have.
   ❏ I am suffering the effects of not reaching this goal.
   ❏ This goal reflects an important value that I hold. Here's how I describe this value: _____

   Other reasons:
   _____
   _____
   _____

After Brain Injury: Tools for Living
A Step-by-Step Guide for Caregivers and Survivors

W 5–2

Using a Graph to Measure Behavior Worksheet

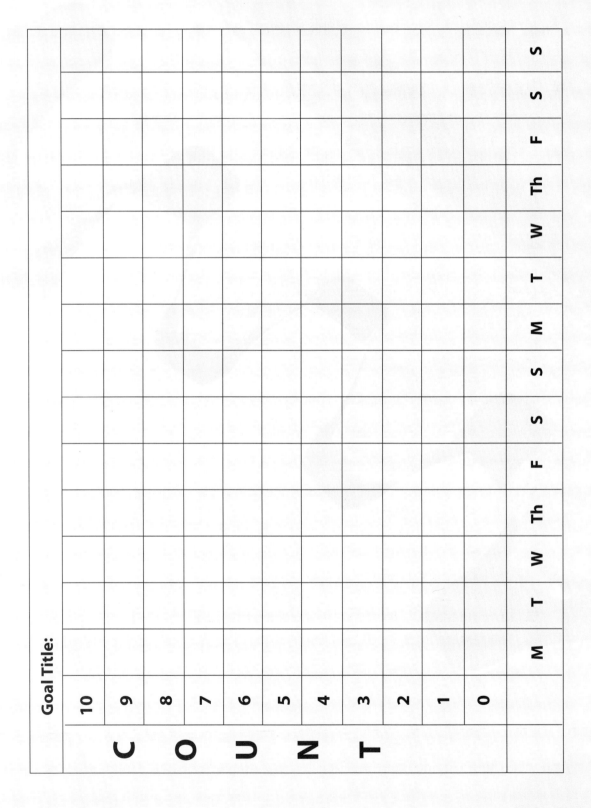

W 5–3

Evaluating Progress Toward My Goal Worksheet

1. My achievable, realistic, measurable goal is: _____
   _____

2. The behavior I am counting and keeping track of at this time is:
   _____

3. Once you have kept track of your progress for several weeks on graphs, make a chart comparing your weekly goal (frequency or interval) to your actual counts (the number of counters you moved in a week).

	Week 1	Week 2	Week 3	Week 4	Week 5
My weekly goal					
My actual count					

4. Look at the chart. Decide whether your progress is:

   ❑ On track. You will keep on doing what is working.
   ❑ Off track. You need to make a change in your goal or in the behavior you're working on.

5. Decide what change to make.

   ❑ Be more realistic. Break this behavior into smaller pieces and then count for the next week.
   ❑ Keep the step, but be kinder to yourself. Try lowering your weekly goal so that you just have to stretch a little to succeed.
   ❑ Ask for help about how to re-shape your goal or your behavior.

6. Plan the changes you need to make. For this, you can use a project-planning worksheet. For ideas, see the Project-Planning Worksheet in Chapter 4.

Rewarding/Celebrating Achievement Worksheet

Make a list of the rewards and celebrations you would like as you achieve your goals.

_____

_____

_____

_____

_____

_____

_____

_____

_____

_____

_____

_____

_____

Weekly Goal Statement About Changing Anger

Identify

The anger problem I am focusing on is:
_____

Describe

My goal meets all these conditions:

- ❏ important
- ❏ conceivable
- ❏ possible
- ❏ controllable
- ❏ measurable
- ❏ has no alternatives

Measure

The counters I'll use are:
_____ (pennies or popcorn kernels)

Evaluate

The method of measurement I'll use is: *(check one)*
❏ frequency (how often)   ❏ interval (how long)

My progress is: ❏ on track ❏ off track
The change I plan to make is:_____
_____

Reward

Review date:_____

I will celebrate my success by:_____
_____

Further Resources Available

Products

After Brain Injury: Tools for Living is a system of educational products designed for growth and healing following a very special type of experience — the trauma resulting from brain injury. The system contains these components:

The Book *After Brain Injury: Tools for Living—A Step-By-Step Guide for Caregivers and Survivors,* written for caregivers and survivors in recovery after brain injury.

The Pocket Guide A small portable notebook of methods and tools condensed from the book *After Brain Injury: Tools for Living,* designed for day-to-day use by survivors.

The TOM System TOM (Time Organization Manager), a binder which caregivers and survivors can use for organizing activities day by day, month by month, and into the future.

Telephone Support Service Available once on a complimentary basis to each purchaser of a component. Caregivers can also arrange for ongoing support as they and their loved ones work through the recovery process. Call 1-866-520-3468.

These components present teaching and learning methods that have proven extremely effective in the recovery process of people with a brain injury and their families. Focusing on psychological recovery — emotional recovery, thinking in new ways and changing behavior — these components recognize the complexity of the recovery process and give caregivers and survivors practical, concrete tools to use throughout recovery and beyond.

All these materials can be ordered online at www.livingafterbraininjury.com or by telephone at 1-866-520-3468.

Internet Resources

These are the consumer-driven associations for caregivers and survivors:

International:	www.internationalbrain.org

USA:	www.biausa.org

UK:	www.headway.org.uk

Australia:	www.headwayvictoria.org.au

Canada:	www.obia.on.ca

www.bcrrc.com

www.brainresources.com

The above organizations will link you to more local resources.

To contact the authors of this book visit:

www.livingafterbraininjury.com

www.brainresources.org

Author Biographies

J. Lynne Mann

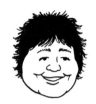

Director and president of her own brain-injury rehabilitation organization since 1983, J. Lynne Mann is a psychologist who originally trained to be a psychotherapist. A person with a disability herself, who resolved to educate the medical specialists about the "living with" aspects of disability, Lynne was quickly drawn into the world of rehabilitation after her training.

Lynne soon found out that almost no Canadian, North American or Continental European phenomenological research had ever been done on the experience of epilepsy. This became her first research in the field of neurological rehabilitation. That research opened a wealth of opportunities to work in Canadian rehabilitation organizations.

Spending her initial career years as a psychological consultant on neurological disabilities and vision impairments, Lynne also became active as a volunteer director of the Manitoba Epilepsy Association. She also became involved with Epilepsy Canada.

Moving to the West Coast, she set up the Adult Vocational Services division of the Vancouver Neurological Centre (now the Centre for Ability), and at the same time consulted to the Centre's residential life-skills teaching program.

Starting her own community-based rehabilitation service in 1983 has led to an exciting and fulfilling career. Lynne has spent 20 years guiding and developing vocational rehabilitation services for persons with brain injury. She developed the first and still unique curriculum for the emotional recovery process from this trauma. Both these services exist within the public sector and the private sector.

In the past two years, Lynne has been working and encouraging her community to develop accredited learning for para-professional community workers. These are workers who either specialize in brain-injury rehabilitation practice or find themselves constantly bumping against their need to know more. As of 2002, core training is now offered through a partnership in training with the Justice Institute of British Columbia.

In the midst of a career life devoted to developing, implementing, and protecting access to services for persons with brain injuries and their families, Lynne also raised a daughter who is an incredible person. Lynne is ever thankful for Lisa, believing that their small family is the best part of her life's work.

Michael Rossiter

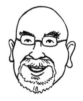

Mike Rossiter contributed a particularly unique combination of skills and expertise to this project.

As the father of a traumatic brain injury survivor, Mike had personal knowledge and experience to offer. In addition, Mike had first-hand experience with advocacy for the brain-injury community, having served as a board member of Brain Associations of BC for three years and as president in his last year. Mike spent much of that time advocating for services and support for survivors and their families. In the process, he met with community leaders and volunteers, as well as with many dedicated service professionals in communities throughout BC.

Mike also brought over 35 years of business experience to this project. In his early working years, Mike returned to college at various times to complete three different, but related, apprenticeships. He has worked directly in or been associated with the print industry for his entire career, and has considerable experience in press, pre-press and graphic design and marketing. For two decades, Mike lived in Northwestern BC where he was the owner and manager of a successful printing business that continues to thrive today. For the past eight years, Mike has been self-employed in the Greater Vancouver area as a graphic designer, working with many clients in the healthcare field.